MEDICAL
FOR HEALTH

A Healer's Guide

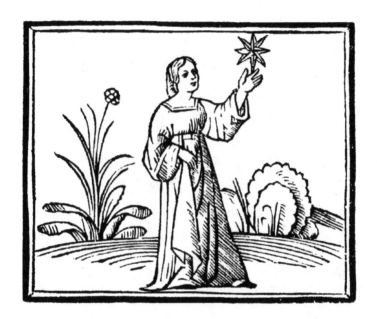

Judith Hill

The Layman's Prequel to:
MEDICAL ASTROLOGY:
A Guide to Planetary Pathology

MEDICAL ASTROLOGY FOR HEALTH PRACTITIONERS:
A Healer's Guide
The Layman's Prequel to: *Medical Astrology:*
A Guide to Planetary Pathology

by Judith Hill

Edited by Amy Faucon
Design, Layout, Cover:
Dawn King Fine Design

STELLIUM
PRESS

Published in 2019 by Stellium Press
Portland, Oregon
Copyright © 2019 by Judith Hill
JudithHillAstrology.com

ISBN: 1-883376-57-2
ISBN: 978-1-883376-57-4

Medical Disclaimer:
The following information is intended for general informational purposes only, and does not constitute medical diagnosis, opinion, or advice. Individuals should always seek their physician's approval before considering any suggestions made in this book. Any application of the information set forth in the following pages is at the reader's discretion, and is his or her sole responsibility.

Illustrations are by Judith Hill unless otherwise specified.
Cover Illustration: "Sybil," from Johann Lichtenberger's *Prognosticatio*, printed in Venice by Nicolas and Dominico dal Jesus de Sandro, 1511.

DEDICATION

For the health practitioner
who senses that something was lost...
that now, must be found.

CONTENTS

LIST OF FIGURES

Preface

MEDICAL ASTROLOGY
FOR Health PRACTITIONERS

The intent of this book is to enable the medical practitioner to readily utilize some essentials of medical astrology, sans the years of experience requisite to the expert. This is possible because, although medical astrology is as complex as any medical field, its "best in show" techniques are reliable enough for basic lay use. Health professionals, in fact, hold a significant advantage over those readers who know astrology but not anatomy, etiology or the process of medical diagnosis! Conversely, the lay reader, armed with a current *Merck Manual* plus a solid understanding of basic medical astrology, outshines most Renaissance physicians. Still, no reader should be mislead into thinking that a few hours of study equals full competence! The greatest physician of all is the one whom is a master of both realms. As said the great 17th century herbalist-astrologer Nicholas Culpepper:

"A physician without astrology is like a pudding without fat."

This book is written for all manner of health practitioners and not astrologers, per se, who may find *Medical Astrology, A Guide to Planetary Pathology,* or *Medical Astrology in Action: The Transits of Health* more adapted to their tastes and knowledge base. This present succinct beginner text is for the naturopath, herbalist or clinical physician who needs simple methods that can be readily understood without too much fuss. However, you astrologers will find plenty of delectable material found nowhere else, especially in Chapters 13 and 15.

This basic book introduces a few reliant techniques, distilled from decades of daily personal observation. These select methods are, in my experience, the tools most useful to the healer; and are also easy to learn. The more advanced astrologer will notice many omissions, i.e. case studies, the four elements, transits, "signatures," etc. These and more beginner, mid-level, and advanced techniques are provided in my other texts on this subject as listed in the back of this introductory work.

However, this text includes special sections and perspectives tailor-made for the physician that my former books do not, and are, in fact, wholly unique to astrological literature. For example, Chapter 15: "Doctor-Patient Compatibility," provides essential tips for avoiding medical mishap by first comparing the birth charts of healer and patient. Practitioners all experience happy harmony with some patients and consistent stress with others. Why not significantly reduce your chances of distressed relations or medical error?

The reader may very well be a licensed medical practitioner free to apply these methods as his or her license permits. For those of you who are not licensed to practice medicine, please note that I don't advocate your use of these methods as a medical tool (and, in fact, legally cannot). Still, the study of this field is well worth your time, and supremely enriching to your medical knowledge base. What you learn herein comprises a substantial part of the original Western medical system, in use by licensed Western physicians until the late seventeenth century. Astrology, herbalism and patient evaluation (urine, tongue, pulse, voice, pallor, etc.) formed the triune base of the ancient technique.

For three centuries now, the foreign sounding language and strange symbols of astrology have blocked off the ears of acceptance within the establishment medical community.

This was not always the case! Throughout the ancient, medieval, and Renaissance worlds, medical astrology was a prominent and essential tool of era physicians, who typically were master astrologers and superb herbalists. In fact, European physicians were required to pass their university astrology exams in order to obtain their medical licenses until 1666. If today's physicians only knew what they were missing! *(See the doctor's quote, end of next page.)*

Two adjacent years shine as historically pivotal towards the influx of this system throughout Europe. The Spanish Inquisition of 1492 and the fall of Constantinople in 1493 sent Greek and Jewish physicians scrambling throughout Europe, carrying their remarkable craft with them. The flower of a conflated medical-astrology-herbalism blossomed in late Renaissance England, with the seminal works of both Nicholas Culpepper and Joseph Blagrave.

The roots of this craft are more ancient still, having been born, weaned and teethed in ancient Greece with rivulets of influence from Egyptian, Babylonian and Hebrew sources. Medical Astrology flourished in the Golden Age of Islam (8th-14th centuries). Practitioners owe a great debt to the Arabs and Jews of this time who preserved, polished, improved, and documented this system in the scholastic centers of Spain and other Islamic centers of the period.

I'm always bemused at the enthusiasm with which today's Western healers accept and adopt traditional Chinese Medicine (TCM) and Ayurveda, while remaining seemingly blind to their own similar and equally venerable system. The culpability lies with the European scientists and "new" physicians of the 18th century, who set about crushing and besmirching their own medical heritage and those who dared practice it.

Their goals at the time were certainly not all bad: stamp out superstition; replace unsanitary and unproven medical practices with scientific methods; and improve knowledge of the body. However, they also endeavored to crush the competition; make more money for themselves by monopolizing medical practice and education; and last but not least, suppress female healers. This last trend began far earlier. In 1421, physician Gilbert Kymer and colleagues petitioned Parliament to ban women from practicing medicine!

Regardless of their staunchest efforts, this remarkable medical system never died, but continued in underground use amongst maverick, and sometimes genius physicians, e.g. Dr. William Davidson, and Howard Leslie Cornell. M.D., L.L.D., D.A., (quoted below), to name but a few. Nevertheless, this astonishingly useful system struggles along, largely ignored. I've endeavored throughout my life to help reinstate this profoundly useful knowledge to its rightful place in Western medical practice.

Microscopes and CAT scans offer new vision into the body and etiological processes but can neither see into the vibrational patterns behind disease manifestation, nor time surgery, treatment, convalescence, or potential death. Herein this lies the supreme value of medical astrology. Healers who diligently observe the simple methods provided in this book may find their reward to be well beyond their imaginings.

In my own practice I found Astrology of inestimable value in diagnosing my cases, and to quickly determine the seat of the disease in the patient, how long they have been sick and ailing, and to form a reasonably accurate prognosis.

– Howard Leslie Cornell, *M.D., L.L.D., D.A.*, 1933,
Author, *The Encyclopedia of Medical Astrology*

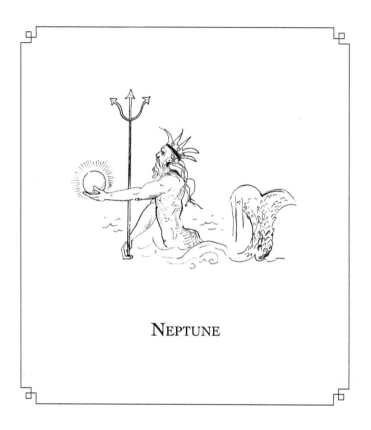

NEPTUNE

Chapter 1
WHAT MEDICAL ASTROLOGY CAN DO FOR YOU

Medical astrology is, above all else, useful. The birth map and current transits provide the healer with practical insight and information not readily available through other means. In effect, the natal chart is a type of microscope that sees into the energetic patterns of the body, and the timing, duration and location of the changes within that vessel.

Having myself performed multiple double-blind tests on the assessment of disease based solely on the horoscope, allow me to vouch for the efficacy of this ancient art. Dr. H. L. Cornell, Dr. William Davidson, Joseph Blagrave, and many other physicians and herbalists down the centuries have staunchly vouched for the veracity of this science.

Short List of Practical Applications
These are not listed in any particular order of importance.
1) Defining type, amount and strength of the patient's innate vital force.
2) Selecting safe surgery dates.
3) Find the seat of chronic disease.
4) Identifying the seat of inflammation.
5) Diagnosing the cause of mysterious symptoms.
6) Comprehending adjunct causes contributive to a disease process.
7) Assisting with fertility and conception.
8) Selecting dates for cesarean section.
9) Knowing when to release a patient from the hospital.

10) Identifying length of illness and mortal potential.
11) Assessing Doctor-Patient harmony / disharmony.
12) Selecting appropriate herbs or treatment.
13) Identifying a patient's innate weaknesses and strengths.
14) Assessing etiological category:
    Is the disease is of physical, psychological or supernatural origin?
15) Understanding the patient's needs.
16) Provides best times for: herbal planting, harvest, decoction and administering
17) Alert you as to when a problem is far more dangerous than you would otherwise know.
18) Determining the onset of menarche, menopause, etc.
19) Selecting the right surgeon.
20) Being alert to individual patient idiosyncrasy and reaction.
21) Being prepared for collective health trends.

Chapter 2
THE TESTIMONY OF PHYSICIANS

TESTIMONY OF DR. WILLIAM DAVIDSON

The following three remarkable quotes are from Dr. William Davidson, physician and medical astrologer, extracted from his *Introduction to Medical Astrology*, third edition, 1978, edited by Helen Ramsey and published by The Astrological Bureau in Monroe, N.Y.

An expert looking at a phonograph record can tell you a great deal, by means of the microscope, about the hills and grooves and what they will produce. The expert astrologer looking at a horoscope can tell what kind of music or disharmony those forces will bring about into the body. So the first thing we must remember is that behind chemistry is force...

Astrology confirms the facts of life. Your horoscope is the graphic representation of the forces that vitalize and maintain your body—hence it is the master key to your physical health and physical idiosyncrasies no less than to the peculiarities and individualities of character....

Almost every disease has its "pseudos". More than that, there are many diseases which have very different types, and to differentiate these types is imperative if you are going to be successful in practice. You can tell in the twinkling of an eye if you use astrology; to the doctor, it gives great insight. The quickness, the speed of it is unbelievable; it's like reading a piece of music. After all, that's what a horoscope is: it's a music of the soul projected into the body....

TESTIMONY OF HOWARD LESLIE CORNELL, M.D., D.A.

...Physicians and Healers should lay aside their prejudices, and investigate Astrology, prove it by observation, and when they do, I feel sure they will give it its rightful place in their Schools and Colleges of Healing, and in their daily practices among their patients. In my own practice, I found Astrology of inestimable value in diagnosing my cases, and to quickly determine the seat of the disease in the patient, how long they have been sick and ailing, and to form a reasonably accurate prognosis....

...In the Fall of 1918, after many years of active Practice in Medical work in this Country, and in India, I gave up the practice of Medicine and moved my family to Los Angeles, and have lived here ever since, and given my whole time to Astrology, Writing and the preparation of Star Maps, Horoscopes and Astrological Health Readings for people all over the World. When this Encyclopaedia is out, circulated and established, it is my plan to make a World Lecture Tour, and speak before the various Healing Centers and Schools in the U.S.A. and other Nations, and to make an effort to have the various Faculties make Medical Astrology one of the required studies for their students who are aspiring to be Healers....

From H. L. Cornell's "Foreword" to his renowned work: *The Encyclopaedia of Medical Astrology*, March 21st, 1933, Third Revised Edition, 1972, Published jointly by Llewellyn Publications, St. Paul, Minnesota and Samuel Weiser, Inc., NYC; available through Astrological Classics.

TESTIMONY OF DR. EUGEN JONAS

"...The results of my research and astrological calculations surprised even me—notably that the discovery of the sex of the embryo depends upon the Moon and that bodies in the solar system

can affect the viability of the newborn child...at first I regarded these things as fantastic and I could not bring myself to believe in their truth. However, my observations and examinations running into thousands of cases in the gynecological clinic in Bratislava showed me that the more obstetric cases I studied, the more exact the astronomical calculations I carried out, the more the results showed me the existence of a hitherto unknown law of nature."

Dr. Eugen Jonas, Chief of the Psychiatric Out-Patient Clinic of Nove Zamky District Institute of Public Health in Czechoslavakia (1968), became director of the Astra Nitra Research Center in Nitra. He is renowned for discoveries related to the astrological influences on timing of conception and conceived gender.

TESTIMONY OF JOSEPH BLAGRAVE (1610-1679), GREAT RENAISSANCE HERBALIST, MEDICAL ASTROLOGER & MEDICAL DIARIST

...For without some knowledge in Astronomy, one can be no Astrologer; and without knowledge in Astrology, one can be no Philosopher, and without Knowledge both in Astrology and Philosophy, one can be no good Physician and whosoever desires to make practice, either in the Astrological or Chymical way of Physick...must build and rely upon these five substantial Pillars following, without which, there can be no admirable cures done or wonders wrought in this noble Art of Physick....

Extract from "An Introductory Preface to The Reader," Blagrave's *Astrological Practice of Physick*, 1671; Reprinted by Astrological Classics, The Astrology Center of America, 2010; Edited and reprinted by the late great publisher William R. "Dave" Roell.

Chapter 3
LET'S GET STARTED

Know the Symbols for the Signs and Planets

You probably have heard of "astrological signs" and are aware that your child or spouse was born in one of them, or that Uncle Joe is a Taurus. It is less commonly known that each zodiac governs a distinct bodily region. Physically, the twelve signs comprise Twelve Body Zones: Aries, Taurus, Gemini, Cancer, Leo, Virgo, Libra, Scorpio, Sagittarius, Capricorn, Aquarius and Pisces. You will learn all about this in Chapter 4: "Zodiacal Human." Because of their preeminence to medical astrology, I've chosen to capitalize "Body Zones," and assign them by number to "their" sign.

When your patient was born, each planet was in one of the twelve signs. The healer must learn in what sign each of their patient's natal (birth) planets lives, especially Saturn!

To know the zodiac sign anyone's Saturn was posited in at birth, you must 1) obtain your patient's birth date and year, and 2) learn how to discover in what sign Saturn, and the planets stood on that special day. The chart on the next page will teach you the symbols of the planets and signs. Learn these symbols, or keep the chart handy.

If you already know how to obtain a birth chart, and find the signs of the Sun, Moon and planets in that birth chart, great, you can skip right to Chapter 4. For those of you who don't, the next paragraph explains how to obtain this information.

What You Will Need To Use This Book

You will need to obtain a copy of the patient's birth chart. If this is untenable, then all you need is their birth day and year, and either an "ephemeris" inclusive of their birth year,

---

Planetary and Sign Symbols

Planets	*Signs*
Sun ☉	Aries ♈
Moon ☽	Taurus ♉
Mercury ☿	Gemini ♊
Venus ♀	Cancer ♋
Mars ♂	Leo ♌
Jupiter ♃	Virgo ♍
Saturn ♄	Libra ♎
Uranus ♅	Scorpio ♏
Neptune ♆	Sagittarius ♐
Pluto ♇	Capricorn ♑
North Lunar Node ☊	Aquarius ♒
South Lunar Node ☋	Pisces ♓
Pars Fortuna ⊗	

---

or access to a chart-calculating website. Although a complete chart requires an accurate birth time and birth place too, I realize that this patient data is often difficult or embarrassing to request.

Alternately, you may work in climate where patients eagerly push their birth charts into your hands! Fortunately, for most of the beginner's skills presented in this book, your patient's birth date and year will suffice to discover the sign of Saturn, so essential to know! The birth date will also serve to establish the signs of the Sun, and every planet except the fast moving Moon, or that rare planet situated on a cusp between two signs. For those, we do need the time and place of birth.

For example, except in rare cases, finding Saturn, and thus, the "seat of disease," requires only a birth date and year. This makes it easy for the complete beginner to dig right in! Any exceptions to this are noted in this text. For instance, the Moon changes signs every two and a half days and may require an exact birth time to know for certain what sign she tenants at birth.

I am not advocating sloppy astrology, *au contraire*. Let it be known that it takes decades to master medical astrology! The intent of this basic layman's text is to introduce a few extremely fruitful methods for immediate use to medical professionals.

Serious students will of course, endeavor to obtain a truly accurate birth chart. For this, you will also need to obtain the patient's birthplace and time, including any variations for daylight savings.

Some chart calculating websites will list the names of the signs and planets of a chart in plain English. Beautiful.

However, with the help of our symbols chart, it's easy enough to learn to read an "ephemeris of planetary motion" for yourself. This skill will empower you to look up anyone's essential Saturn and Mars positions in your new handy pocket guide (the ephemeris).

There are many websites that will teach you how. Just google: "How to read an ephemeris." My favorite site is "skyscript" at:
http://skyscript.co.uk/ephemeris.html

Or, read the tips in the addendum: "How to read an ephemeris."

Step By Step

First and foremost, you need to be able to recognize the simple symbols for the twelve signs, Sun, Moon, planets, Lunar Nodes. The chart on the previous page is provided for your ready use.

This is a new language and takes a little practice. Some symbols you already know! The Sun and Moon look exactly like they should! Venus and Mars are still in standard medical use for symbolizing "female" and "male." First learn to recognize Saturn, and then, to know the sign he was in on the day that your patient was born. Now, you already hold a master key to medical astrology!

Next, you will need to meet traditional "Zodiacal Man." This is his traditional name. However, if you prefer, feel free to substitute Zodiacal Woman or Zodiacal Human (he doesn't care). In this manner, you will know what bodily regions are governed by which zodiac sign (next chapter). Once you recognize your symbols and the 12 Body Zones of Zodiacal Man, you are ready to begin using basic medical astrology.

Important! The health idiosyncrasies described in this book for planets, Sun, Moon and the twelve signs are not givens. Many people of all signs go through life in perfect health! Descriptions are intended for the medical professional's greater awareness, and not for self-suggestion by those curiously reading about their own planet and sign positions. *(See medical disclaimer on copyright page.)*

This book is not intended as a guide for negative self-suggestion, but rather as an assistant to healers working with already manifested symptoms.

Astrologers should note that it requires "three testimonies" for even the possibility of sure physical manifestation. Planets and signs do not always express themselves physically in terms of health maladies.

Chapter 4

ZODIACAL MAN (HUMAN)

Renaissance physicians were highly intelligent persons, experts in herbalism, and master astrologers. They relied on an ancient device termed "Zodiacal Man" as a primary diagnostic and treatment timing tool. For some concerns, it remains unsurpassed to this day!

Hopefully, you now know your symbols and how to use a basic ephemeris. Now, you will need to familiarize yourself with "Zodiacal Man," the medical chart that was a mainstay of every physician's and surgeon's office until around 1666. For this purpose, I've designed two modern-looking zodiacal men (readily interchangeable with zodiacal women for those who prefer the female form).

These figures are more complete than their medieval predecessors, (who failed to show the posterior) and hopefully, less gruesome. An example from the Renaissance is also provided, guts exposed. The problem with early models is that they do not show the back, and also neglect some finer details.

Please don't assume this system disappeared! Zodiacal Man has continued on in use with practitioners of medical astrology; (including many modern-day renegade physicians) throughout the centuries and remains widely popular today, and useful.

Zodiacal Man starts at the top of the head with the first sign, Aries, Body Zone 1. As we proceed down the body, we likewise proceed through the signs in the 12 Body Zones. The cycle ends with the last sign, Pisces, ruling Zone 12, the feet.

This is easy to comprehend if you envision a circle of twelve divisions (the Solar year) that is converted into a single vertical line (the human body). In this manner, the human body reflects the circle of the year, the twelve zodiac signs, and the 360 astrological degrees. This is the basis for Zodiacal Man and his twelve, sign governed Body Zones.

Zodiacal Human: Sign-Body Correlation

Note: The use of numbered "Body Zones," in lieu of traditional zodiac sign names, is my own device created to assist the medically inclined non-astrologer to understand (and *use*) the system with less prejudice.

It is hardly possible to list all body organs here. For individual vessels, vertebrae, and muscles, please refer to Dr. H. L. Cornell's *Encyclopedia of Medical Astrology*.

In medical astrology we have general system rulerships, followed by more precise designations. For instance, Sagittarius (Zone 9) rules the arterial circulation in general, although vessels also come under the influence of their residence zone. Medical astrology is an evolving science. To date, not all body parts have been assigned their corresponding planetary and sign influences, e.g. the individual brain hemispheres and blood constituents.

Aries – Body Zone 1: Top of the head, (cranium) eyes, motor centers of brain, upper jaw and teeth, some head nerves; and the adrenal glands (shared with Libra and Mars). The entire brain in general is strongly influenced by Aries, along with the Sun, Moon and Mercury. The sense of sight is under the province of this sign, in concert with the Sun and Moon.

Taurus – Body Zone 2: Lower head, lower teeth and jaw, ears; tonsils (shared with Scorpio); tongue, vocal chords (shared with Venus and Mercury); salivary glands, lower brain, hypothalamus, pons, medulla (shared with Aries), thyroid (shared with Uranus, Venus, and Mercury), neck, cervical nerves and vertebra, neck muscles, gullet, throat, upper esophagus, swallowing reflex, epiglottis, jugular vein, carotid arteries, and atlas and axis bones.

The sense of hearing is strongly influenced by this sign, in concert with Aries, Mercury, Saturn and Mars.

Gemini – Body Zone 3: Bronchial tubes, upper lungs, inspiration (as opposed to respiration), shoulders, clavicle, scapula, arms, radius and ulna, arms, and hands. The wrists and forearms are shared with Leo. Bodily capillaries, speech centers of brain, peripheral afferent nerves and coordination, and the tubes of the body in general (each sign co-governing the capillaries and tubes within its Zone).

Cancer – Body Zone 4: Lower lung, breast, stomach, lower esophagus, meninges and pleura, thoracic duct, rib cage, sternum; scapula (shared with Gemini); elbow, armpit, pancreas (shared with Virgo); diaphragm. Cancer exerts influence over temperature regulation, the hypothalamus and thalamus; posterior pituitary (with Jupiter); gums; the umbilicus (Hill, Cornell says Virgo). Some authors allot all hollow bodily cavities to Cancer, including the eyes sockets and cheeks. This author is not in full agreement. Cancer and Pisces both hold a significant rulership over the lymphatic fluid and nodes.

Some say that Cancer rules the bone marrow, although this complex substance certainly involves more rulerships. Cancer greatly influences female fertility, lactation, and the uterus when pregnant. This sign has a considerable influence over the mucus membrane and the general moisture level of the internal tissue. A mucus producing sign.

Leo – Body Zone 5: Heart, aorta, dorsal vertebrae, general spinal alignment, spinal sheaths; and the gallbladder (shared with Capricorn, Saturn, and Mars). Governs the longissimus, lattissimus dorsi, transversalis and heart muscles. The forearms and wrists are shared with Gemini.

Virgo – Body Zone 6: Upper intestinal organs, liver (shared with Jupiter with influence from Leo and Cancer); pancreas and spleen (shared with Cancer); upper intestine; ascending colon (shared with Scorpio); immune system (shared with Pisces); automatic nervous system, and sympathetic nerves. The portal circulation (co-ruled with the signs and planets that govern the arteries and veins in general). The fingers (shared with Gemini and Mercury).

Libra – Body Zone 7: Kidneys, ovaries, lumbar spine, buttocks (shared with Sagittarius) sense of balance, acid-alkaline balance, salt and fluid balance, and adrenal glands (shared with Mars and Aries). Cornell places the buttocks themselves (but not the hips) under Libra, although these are usually assigned to Sagittarius (Nauman), with influence from Scorpio (the sacrum and anus is under Scorpio, and the coccyx under Scorpio and Sagittarius).

Scorpio – Body Zone 8: Excretory system (shared with Mars), nose, bladder and bladder sphincter, cervix, neck of uterus, (with Cancer and the Moon, Scorpio greatly influences the uterus), genitals, urethra, colon, prostate, rectum, anus, sweat glands, sacrum, brim of pelvis. Tonsils (co-ruled with Taurus).

Sagittarius – Body Zone 9: Hips, thighs, femurs, the arterial circulation in general (with Jupiter), but most specifically the external iliac, femoral and sacral arteries; with significant influence over the vena sacra, iliac and great saphenous veins (with Venus and Aquarius). This sign rules over the lower spinal nerves. The buttocks (shared with Libra and Scorpio).

This sign has a significant influence on the coordination processes of the central nervous system (CNS), and the motor nerves; and the voluntary muscular system (shared with Mars and Aries). Sagittarius and Scorpio both influence the sacrum and coccyx. Sagittarius also governs the breath's expiration, in partnership with its polar opposite sign Gemini, the sign of inspiration.

Capricorn – Body Zone 10: Knees, patella; the skin, ligaments, tendons, and cuticles of the body in general. This sign has a significant influence (with Saturn) over the entire skeletal system, joints and bones. Capricorn is noted to govern the anterior pituitary (with Jupiter).

Aquarius – Body Zone 11: Ankles, shins; venous system (shared with Venus); the oxygenation of the blood (shared with Gemini); general quality of blood, and the little known electrical system of the body. This sign strongly influences the spinal nerves (with Sagittarius). Some authors cite the rods and cones of the eye as under the dominion of this sign. Cornell allots "the pyramidal tract of the spinal cord" to this sign. Aquarius and Sagittarius both greatly influence the spinal nerves, (whereas Leo governs the spinal sheaths).

Pisces – Body Zone 12: Feet, toes, lymphatic system (with Cancer), parasympathetic nervous system, sleep, supernatural etiologies, and subconsciously induced health issues. The extracellular matrix, the lymphatic system in general (with Cancer ruling the thoracic duct), and cellular hydration. Pisces influences the cecum and duodenum (shared with Virgo), and influences the porousness of the intestinal tract, intestinal mucous levels, and the absorption of nutrients through the intestinal wall.

This sign is highly receptive and fertile. Pisces and Cancer are the most mucous producing signs. Pisces appears to govern the general coordination (or lack of) the ductless glands. It is interesting to note that Pisces' planetary ruler, Jupiter, was said by Edgar Cayce to govern the pituitary gland. This gland is also strongly linked to the signs Cancer (posterior) and Capricorn (anterior).

Organs and Ductless Glands: Planet and Sign Associations

The planets rule many organs, glands, and physical processes on their own, and / or share these with various signs. This material is addressed in my more advanced text: *Medical Astrology: Your Guide to Planetary Pathology.* Remember, this current work is a beginner's text created exclusively for quick use by healers, who are not always astrologers, per se.

Don't be confused should you encounter various planet / sign co-rulerships of bodily organs. This is normal, and rather like two brothers sharing one house. Generally speaking, the 12 zodiac signs rule the 12 Body Zones, with the planets governing the internal organs…but there is considerable overlap.

Example: The sign Cancer (Body Zone 4) governs the stomach, ribcage, lower lung, thoracic duct and the breasts. The Moon co-governs the stomach and breast! Those of you who study the charts of sufferers of stomach and breast issues will find these co-rulerships valid.

Although there are many extant opinions on the planetary rulerships attributed to the ductless glands (Cornell, Nauman, Davidson *et al.*), this author is fascinated by the assignments given by the great medical psychic Edgar Cayce:

Mercury – pineal   Saturn – the gonads
Venus – thymus   Uranus – thyroid
Mars – adrenals   Neptune – leyden
Jupiter – pituitary

These two illustrations *(Figure 1 & 2)* more clearly depict the 12 Body Zones than do Renaissance models. The first drawing shows the anterior view. The organs located within these zones share rulership with various planets. *(See Chapter 10.)*

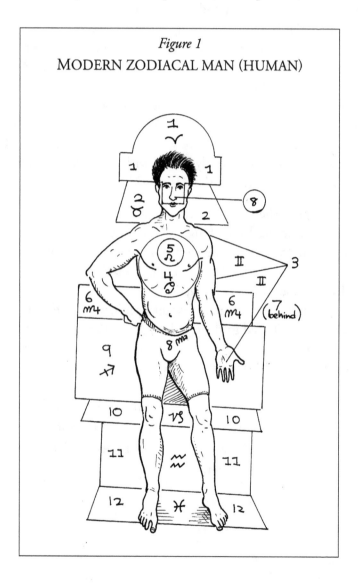

Figure 1
MODERN ZODIACAL MAN (HUMAN)

Lateral view, exposing the Leo and Libra regions not visible in the old frontal views. The organs located within these zones share rulership with various planets. *(See Chapter 10.)*

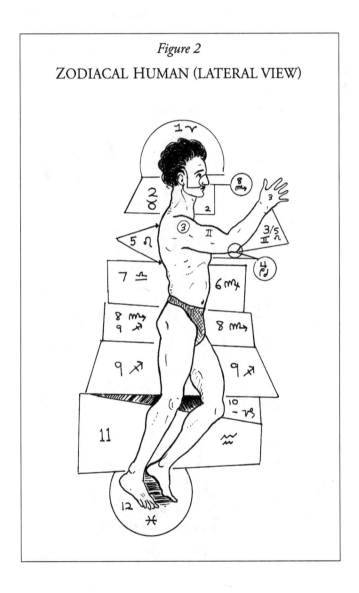

Figure 2

ZODIACAL HUMAN (LATERAL VIEW)

Figure 3

HOMO SIGNORUM – THE MAN OF SIGNS

From Johann Regiomantus' *Kalendarius Teutsch,* printed by Johann Sittich, Augsburg, 1512. Also known as "Zodiacal Man," similar images were displayed in Renaissance surgeon's offices. The use of the Moon's transits through its four phases and the twelve signs was essential knowledge for the selection of safe surgery dates.

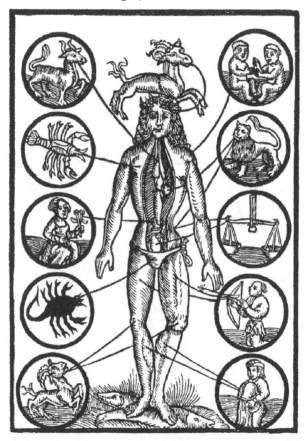

Klarhayt der zeit beffert alle Laß tag

Chapter 5

SATURN: THE KEY TO CHRONIC DISEASE

Saturn: The Seat of Chronic Illness

Action of Saturn: Cold, Dry, Slow, Restrictive

Know the sign of your patient's Saturn!

Saturn's zodiac sign position in your patient's birth chart will indicate where their body tends to be cold, tight, tense, slow, restricted, or hypo functioning. This area lacks oxygen or blood flow. Toxins amass. Disease process begins here. Saturn is the foremost seat of chronic disease.

You don't need to be an advanced medical astrologer to use this key. Go for it!

Armed with Saturn's sign at the birth of your patient, you are possessed of a medical key as precious as pure gold. Find the Saturn's natal sign in your patient's birth chart. Next, correlate this sign to the Body Zone it rules. Now, put on your puzzle-solving thinking cap.

Something within or about Saturn's bodily zone may, over time, be the seat of disease. Why? Saturn indicates that this region is astrally "cold" and inclined to oxygen deprivation, restricted circulation, or inadequate nutrition. This same region becomes "tight" hardened, or constricted. Tissue may dry, or tumors develop. Toxins amass.

Additionally, the structure of this Body Zone may be too small or structurally misaligned or stenotic. This is because Saturn rules the bones, the hard structures of the body.

Saturn's natal sign placement has long been held to be the source of most chronic disorders. Saturn's cold ray also restricts the Body Zones governed by the zodiac signs located opposite to the sign he tenants, and also those signs positioned at 90°

distant to him in the horoscope. You can find these opposite and squared sign pairings in Chapter 15. However, this is more advanced and may confuse the layman. Beginners need concern yourself only with Saturn's natal sign placement. He is felt most strongly here!

Traditionally, Saturn's maladies are treated with primarily warming remedies; and secondly, moistening, depending on presenting symptoms and the element of Saturn's sign. This information is of inestimable worth to the healer! Chronic disease takes time to develop and can be preempted in many cases.

We have not discussed Saturn by element in this book, that being more advanced material. For now, his Body Zone (sign) will suffice. The examples that follow will clarify how the system works. The logic is mechanical, as in: A+B=C.

Example 1: (See *Figure 4, next page.*) Perhaps a patient is suffering from a chronic cough. You have found that they were born when cold Saturn was in Body Zone 3, Gemini: the sign of the upper lung and bronchial tubes. This suggests "cold" or "dry" bronchitis, with serious or chronic potential. The herbalist would consider the warming expectorants and relaxing demulcents specific to the lungs.

Do you see how very different this causative energy is from similar symptoms presenting for a patient with Mars in Gemini? (See *Figure 6, page 28.*) Mars would indicate dry heat, infection, or inflammation of the upper respiratory track. The healer would instead, opt for cooling expectorants and relaxing demulcents! Let's return to Saturn.

Saturn in Gemini suggests deficient respiration and blocked tubules. Respiration is slowed, and sub oxygenation sets in. Conversely, Mars says excessive excretion, and raw inflammation. To use medical astrology, the Western physician

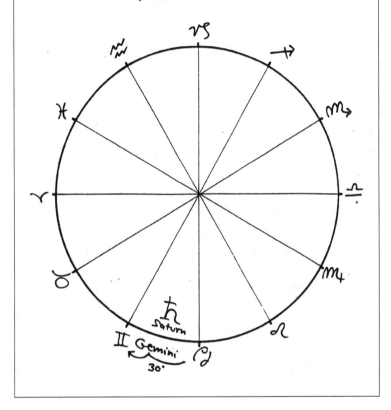

Figure 4

SATURN IN GEMINI

Note: Saturn's House Position in this Figure is arbitrary. He could be in any one of the twelve houses (divisions).

must learn to think energetically. Let's consider this approach in more depth.

To reiterate: **Saturn is cold, slow, dry, astringent / Mars is hot, fast, dry, expulsive.**

Ayurvedic physicians and naturopaths already know the variety of maladies that manifest from excess cold-dry versus hot-dry. All you need to do now is to learn the energies of each planet and then reason out how these energies might express themselves physically through each of the traditional 12 Body Zones listed for Zodiacal Human.

Example 2: *(See Figure 5, next page.)*

Let's drive this point home. Perhaps you have a patient who is suffering protracted fatigue but cannot determine the source. You observe that your patient was born with Saturn in Leo. Zodiacal Man tells us that Leo is Body Zone 5: heart, aorta, upper back, spinal sheaths, and gall bladder. As a physician, you are in good stead to consider all the possibilities that this might suggest.

In fact, you have a singular advantage over any astrologers who do not share your medical training and experience!

Saturn in Leo suggests any (and more) of the following potential conditions may be contributing to the symptoms of chronic fatigue: restricted heart vessels, lack of oxygen to the heart muscle, organic heart problem, heart failure, deficient bile, blocked gall ducts, misaligned vertebrae. The physician must now apply this astrological clue to the patient's symptom of fatigue.

If this route is not productive, check out the Body Zone of the patient's Lunar South Node (the bringer of fatigue), or Neptune. Their actions will be discussed in upcoming chapters.

As Dr. Davidson testified, you can see so very much "in the twinkling of an eye."

The more advanced practitioner can narrow each Body Zone down further into thirty traditional segments ("degrees"), each correlating with a distinct bodily region! However, knowing your general region is good enough for now.

Knowing the natal sign position of a patient's Saturn can help healers preempt future problems by warming,

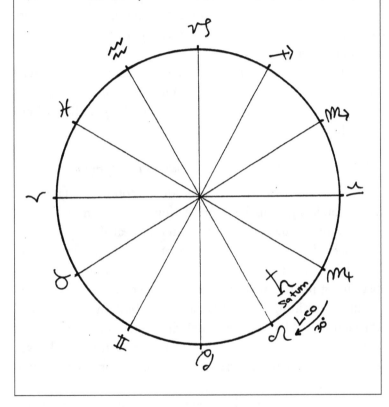

Figure 5

SATURN IN LEO

Note: Saturn's House Position in this Figure is arbitrary. He could be in any one of the twelve houses (divisions).

moistening, relaxing, and increasing circulation in this Body Zone!

Saturn's sign-related maladies per sign, are already detailed in *Medical Astrology: A Guide to Planetary Pathology*, (and many other books as well). Also, the simple examples given above and following will show you how the system works.

Medical practitioners who think astrologically don't need prompting lists because they already know their anatomy and etiology. Simply apply the thoughts: "cold, dry, slow, tight, impeded, deprived, toxic, or skeletal" to the Body Zone (sign) of your patient's birth Saturn as shown by Zodiacal Man. Now, imagine all of the relevant chronic maladies that proceed from these causes, over time, in that bodily region. For fun, let's give another classic example.

Saturn in Body Zone 7 (kidneys), is famous for mineral deposits in the kidney tubules. Dr. Davidson insisted this caused the chronic headaches experienced by sufferers born with this natal Saturn position.

When a Cold Pattern (Saturn) Produces Hot Symptoms (Mars)

In rare cases, cold Saturn can produce a condition of trapped, slowly building heat, i.e. "smoldering." He accomplishes this by preventing the rising up or escape of heat through normal channels. This is more likely to occur when Saturn is in an "Earth" sign: Taurus, Virgo or Capricorn. You often note this placement in arthritic conditions and overheated liver.

In determining if you have a case of building heat created through cold blockage, consider the patient's symptoms first and next check if they were born with Saturn in Earth sign, or otherwise related to the involved Body Zone. Green light soothes this issue!

Saturn is typically quite drying, especially in Fire and Earth signs. However, in Water signs Cancer, Scorpio and Pisces, he can actually trap water, producing torpor and damp toxicity. This is all so interesting and subtle! For now, attend to the basic meanings.

Approach to Treatment for Saturn's Maladies
(for licensed medical practitioners)

Should symptoms present in the Body Zone of natal Saturn, consider remedies and treatments that are relaxing, warming, stimulating, nourishing, oxygenating, moistening, and toxin-excreting. You may need to open the excretory channels of Saturn's natal Body Zone. Typically, these are "constipated."

For example, with natal Saturn in Pisces, aka Body Zone 12, the lymph clearance faculty is typically slowed. Also consider the possibility that skeletal misalignment is occurring somewhere within Saturn's natal Body Zone; or maybe he suggests some other restrictive type organic structural problem. Now you are thinking astrologically! Once you gain confidence, you can progress to more advanced energy treatment methods (detailed in my other texts).

Fun Fact: Each planet antidotes one of various excesses of Saturn. Conversely, Saturn balances the excesses of every planet! Where would we be without his form-defining role?

Saturn is dark / Sun is light (photons, sunlight)

Saturn dries / Moon moistens

Saturn concentrates mind / Mercury quickens mind

Saturn is dry and tight / Venus is demulcent and relaxing

Saturn is cold and slow / Mars is hot and stimulating

Saturn is constrictive and depressed / Jupiter is expansive, and joyful

Saturn is grounded / Uranus is electrical

Saturn is astringent, consolidating and Earthy / Neptune is leaky, diffusive and ethereal

Saturn disciplines feeling / Pluto produces extreme feelings

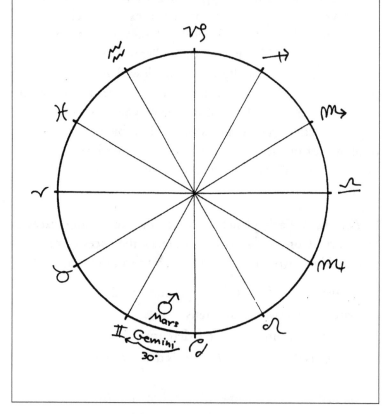

Figure 6

MARS IN GEMINI

Note: Mars' House Position in this Figure is arbitrary. He could be in any one of the twelve houses (divisions).

Chapter 6
MARS: THE SEAT OF INFLAMMATION
Mars: The Cause of Acute Ailments

Action of Mars: Hot, Dry, Stimulating, Excreting

Know the sign of your patient's Mars!

Mars' zodiac sign position in your patient's birth chart suggests their personal Body Zone most inclined towards heat, hyperfunction, inflammation, infection, invasion, infection, excretion, wounds, burns and accidents. Mars penetrates inwardly (wounds, insemination). He also penetrates outwardly (excretion).

If you cannot calculate or read charts, then learn to use an ephemeris of daily planetary motion *(see Addendum)*.

Mars suggests tendencies within his natal sign (Body Zone) towards inflammation, excretion, acidosis, infection, itch, skin eruptions, accidents, surgery and bleeding.

Zodiacal Man will now inform you as to the Body Zone indicated by the sign that your patient's Mars tenanted at birth. Something within this body region usually tends towards inflammation at some point in the lifetime.

Example: Perhaps your patient has suffered a persistent cough. You discover she was born with Mars in Body Zone 3, Gemini. Zodiacal Man informs us that Gemini governs the bronchial tubes and upper lungs. *(See Figure 6, facing page.)* You might now consider that Mars' drying astral heat contributes to the cough.

Dry heat can mean a lot of things, and this is where your medical knowledge intervenes. Potentials to consider might be: bronchial infection, pathogenic invasion or entities; dry, inflamed tissue with lack of moist protection; dry, hot asthma, etc.

Mars is also invasive, and therefore indicative of pathogens. As a fighter, Mars can suggest an exaggerated allergic defense.

Conversely, what if Saturn, instead of Mars, was in Gemini? Then consider cold causes, (instead of hot): stricture, hardening, tension, and entrapped toxins as causative to this patient's cough. Both Mars and Saturn bring dryness. However, in some cases, Saturn can trap moisture, creating fluidic stagnation.

As you see, there are many disease candidates for "hot and dry" within any Body Zone. Equally so, there are a wide variety of maladies possible for "cold and dry" within any Body Zone.

Your patient's birth chart helps you quickly narrow down the general seat of the ailment. The combined knowledge of symptoms, anatomy and the natal chart creates insightful physicians. As you obtain more skill, you can learn to divide each Body Zone into their thirty traditional sub-sections (because all signs have thirty "degrees").

Also, you can learn how Saturn and Mars extend their cold and hot influences to other signs on the season wheel. This is heartier fare and is not required to get started. A planet's effect on the sign it tenants at birth is preeminent! Don't get overwhelmed; just get started!

When Mars Produces Hot and Wet Symptoms (instead of hot-dry)

Mars in Cancer, Scorpio and Pisces sometimes tends to hot and wet conditions! Fungal infections, wet rashes and diarrhea are common.

When Hot Produces Cold Symptoms

In rare cases, hot Mars produces cold by throwing off the heat at the periphery (think of shivering produced by fever, or hypothermia.) This is most typical of Mars in Fire signs: Aries, Leo, Sagittarius—especially Aries!

In determining if you have a case of chill produced by rising heat, first note your patient's symptoms, and next check if they were born when Mars was in a Fire sign or otherwise related to the involved bodily region. Green light is useful for balancing hot-cold issues.

Mars Through the 12 Signs (Body Zones)

Mars maladies through all twelve Body Zones (signs) are already fully detailed in *Medical Astrology: Your Guide to Planetary Pathology*. Medical practitioners who think astrologically don't need prompting lists because they already know their etiology and anatomy.

Simply apply the thought: "hot, dry, inflamed, hyper-functioning, burning, acidic, invading, energizing, bleeding, and stimulating" to the Body Zone (zodiac sign) of your patient's birth Mars. Then, consider all the acute maladies that might express themselves over time in that manner, and in that place.

More Examples: Perhaps a patient arrives with natal Mars in Leo. Body Zone 5. *(See Figure 7, next page.)* Automatically, symptoms permitting, you know they may have some tendency toward arterial blood surges, high pulse, aortic dissection, heart attack, stroke, and back or spinal cord injury). This is astrological thinking.

Note: Mars' hot ray also excites the sign opposite to his natal sign and also those signs positioned at 90° and 150° distant on the seasonal wheel. (This is for more advanced astrologers.) You can find the opposite and squared sign pairing listed in Chapter 15. Beginners need only concern themselves with Mars' natal sign placement.

Figure 7

MARS IN LEO

Note: Mars' House Position in this Figure is arbitrary.
He could be in any one of the twelve houses (divisions).

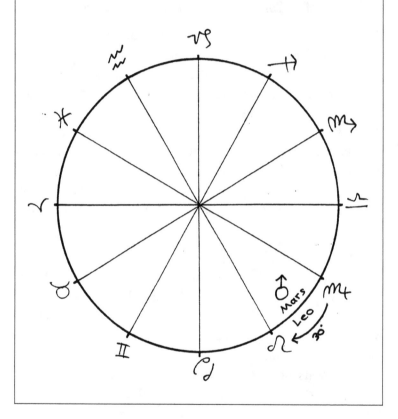

Approach to Treatment for Mars' Maladies
(for licensed medical practitioners)

Should symptoms present in any Body Zone where Mars is found at birth, consider the possibility of infection, bleeding, parasitical or bacterial invasion, or inflammation. Strong excretory responses with fever, biliousness, itch or rash are typical.

Treat with cooling astringents, expectorants or cooling demulcents, as needed. Think alkaline. Strictly avoid hot, drying herbs unless, as in some cases, one must "fetch out fire with fire," but always with the addition of cooling demulcents in the mix. Renaissance master Joseph Blagrave discusses the combining of sympathetic versus antipathetic cures in the exclusive case of Mars, more thoroughly in Blagrave's *Astrological Practice of Physick*. (All other planets are almost always treated with antipathetic cure.)

If Mars is posited in a Water sign (Cancer, Scorpio or Pisces), excess effluvia resulting from infection or hyper excretion may require mopping up! Antibiotics may be required.

Relaxants are helpful for over-stimulation, provided there is no hemorrhage. Pain relief may be in order. Check for issues related to the symptoms that may be linked to any of the following: anemia or problems with red blood cells, bleeding, iron, adrenalin, or testosterone. Test for invading parasites, worms, or bacteria.

Mars induced maladies seldom need excretory assistance. However, under his beams the excretory channels can quickly become overwhelmed! The alterative family of blood and lymph clearing herbs are helpful. Symptoms rule, blended with your knowledge of planetary energetics.

Once you gain confidence, you can progress to more advanced treatment methods (detailed in my other texts).

Knowing the position of a patient's Mars helps the healer preempt future problems by allaying heat and inflammation within this specific Body Zone!

There are many authors besides myself with published disease lists for natal planet placement through the twelve zodiac signs (Nauman, Garrison, *et al.*). Because of so many disease possibilities per planet-sign combination, lists vary! No one author can get it all.

Chapter 7
THE SOUTH LUNAR NODE:
DEFICIENCY, "POWER OUTAGE"

Action of the South Node: Draining, weak, deficient

Know the sign of your patient's South Node.

On the patient's birth date, the sign position of the Lunar South Node will suggest where there is a leak of vital force, weakness, fear, hyper-sensitivity, or insufficiency.

The South Node is also associated with inherited genetic patterns, specifically to the maternal side. Homeopaths might relate this to their concept of "miasm." It's fine to use the shorter term "South Node."

What are the two Lunar Nodes? The Nodes, or "knots" are the two points where Luna's orbit intersects with the earth's orbital path about the Sun, aka the "ecliptic plane". The South Node is the juncture where the Moon intersects this plane moving from North to South, whereas the North Node marks her trajectory from South to North. Luna crosses these points approximately once each, per month.

Solar Eclipses always occur near or conjunct one of the Nodes. Lunar eclipses invariably occur near or conjunct both Nodes.

Together, the Lunar Nodes indicate the directional current of Solar-Lunar forces, that incoming and outflowing tide of energies we know too little about. Traditionally, the Nodes are held in some ways to be more powerful than the planets. In practice, this is true indeed.

As two of the four most reliant precursors of disease, the Lunar Nodes deserve their own special chapters alongside the two traditional "malefics" Saturn and Mars. Knowledge of the Nodes is invaluable to the physician intent on disease prevention!

How to Find the Sign of the South Lunar Node

Find the symbol of the South Node in your patient's chart. If you do not have their chart, then locate their birth date and year in your ephemeris. Now find the South Node on that birth date. Uh-oh, you can't because it's not there?

Many birth charts and most ephemerides list only the symbol for the North Node! This is puzzling, considering the overwhelming importance of the South Node. If you do not see its symbol, then write down the sign of the North Node instead, and use the sign exactly opposite. *(See Opposite Signs chart below.)*

If you are using an ephemeris, be sure to check for any possible sign changes as you move up the column from bottom to top. Once in approximately every one and one-half years, the North Node changes sign during the birth month!

Now you know the sign position of your patient's South Node (again, this is opposite the sign of your patient's North Node). This knowledge gives you an essential key to your patient's health.

OPPOSITE SIGNS / THE SIX POLARITIES

Aries – Libra	Cancer – Capricorn
Taurus – Scorpio	Leo – Aquarius
Gemini – Sagittarius	Virgo – Pisces

Figure 8

FINDING ᴛʜᴇ SOUTH NODE

The South Node will always be found exactly opposite by sign to the sign of the listed North Node.

See the "Opposite Signs" chart. There are six polarities listed. Now, find the sign that you have discovered the natal North Node to tenant. Now find its opposite sign in the chart. This will always be the sign for your patient's all-important natal South Node!

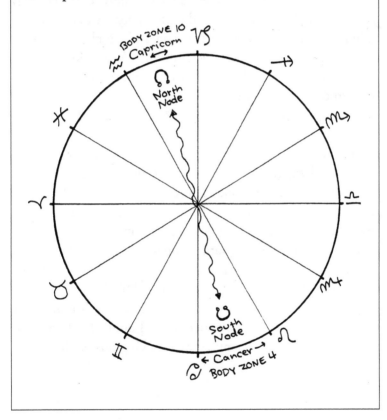

The South Node Through the 12 Signs (Body Zones)

Lists of maladies attributed to the South Node through all twelve signs have been detailed twice in my other books: *Medical Astrology: Your Guide to Planetary Pathology*, and *The Lunar Nodes: Your Key to Excellent Chart Interpretation*, Chapter 13, "The Medical Nodes." *The Lunar Nodes* includes health interpretations for the Nodes in conjunction with all planets.

Medical practitioners who think astrologically don't need prompting lists because they already know their etiology and anatomy! Simply apply the thoughts: "weak, drained, fatigued, deficient, genetic issue, and addiction" to the Body Zone (zodiac sign) of your patient's birth South Node. Then, consider the congenital maladies that might express themselves over time in that manner in that place.

Examples: (See Figure 8, page 37, for Example 1, illustrating South Node in Cancer.) Let us imagine that your patient was born when the South Node was in Cancer, Body Zone 4. This would suggest to you an innate weakness to be found somewhere in Body Zone 4. Perhaps, there is a deficiency in the stomach, breast, lower lung, or elbow; or a tendency toward miscarriage; or insufficient lactation.

Perhaps your patient suffers indigestion. Tests have been inconclusive. You note that the patient's South Node is in Leo, one of the signs known to "rule" the gallbladder. This might suggest a weakly functioning or lazy gallbladder. It is also wise to know the sign of your patient's natal South Node because future problems are preempted by tonifying this bodily zone.

Approach to Treatment

If symptoms agree, these congenital weaknesses in the associated Body Zone can be tonified. As you see, this treatment approach would be quite different than for symptoms manifesting from the North Node, Saturn, or Mars, etc.

However, the South Node is the preeminent indicator of supernatural etiologies, and also, those ailments of purely subconscious origin. These include childhood trauma, paranoia, PTSD, hypochondria, and, for those who believe: disturbing memories arising from previous incarnations.

If symptoms suggest, an investigation of possible supernatural etiology (hexes, possession, etc.) can be fruitful. Ancient and Renaissance physicians wisely utilized a far wider etiological palette than do modern Western physicians.

South Node issues respond well to subtle vibrational remedies: Bach flower essences, homeopathy, musical tones. However, hypnosis and hypnotherapy could be significantly dangerous for the treatment of South Node indicated symptoms, due to the extreme psychic porousness of this indicator. For both the North and South Nodes, genetic and DNA testing may be relevant.

Chapter 8

THE NORTH LUNAR NODE: EXCESS, "POWER SURGE"

Action of the North Node:
Amassing, hardening, impacting, strengthening

Know the sign of your patient's North Node.

What are the Nodes? This answer is detailed at the head of Chapter 7, under "Action of the South Node."

Why is the North Node so important? See the explanation for this too, in the same section.

On the birth date and year of the patient, the sign position of their Lunar North Node may suggest a Body Zone more prone to engorgement, impaction, stroke, hardening, sclerotic processes, swelling, tumor growth, pathogen invasion, or sepsis (if unattended). The North Node is also associated with inherited genetic patterns.

However, the North Node also gives strength, and significantly amplifies the powers of any natal planet sitting next to it in the same zodiac sign! This is called a "conjunction."

Find the birth date of your patient in your ephemeris. Now locate the symbol for the North Node on that birth date at the top menu bar of the ephemeris. If you are using a computerized or preprinted birth chart, find the symbol next to the North Node in the chart's table of planets and signs.

Next, find the Body Zone (zodiac sign) that the natal North Node is in. Its symbol looks just like a horse shoe positioned with the open end at bottom.

Zodiacal Man will tell you the Body Zone ruled by the zodiac sign that your patient's North Node is in. This knowledge provides you with an essential key to your patient's health, so useful in many ways.

Should symptoms present within the Body Zone of your patient's birth North Node, consider that "too much" of something is going on in this region. Often, there is a slow massing of some kind of pressure. Cancer is possible in some cases (rare). Skin conditions are noted.

It is wise to note the sign position (Body Zone) of a patient's birth North Node in order to preempt future problems by reducing pressure, toxin accumulation, or hardening in this bodily zone.

The North Node Through the 12 Signs (Body Zones):

Lists of potential maladies by sign are detailed in *Medical Astrology: A Guide to Planetary Pathology*, and, again in *The Lunar Nodes, Your Guide to Excellent Chart Interpretation*, Chapter 13, "*The Medical Nodes.*"

Medical practitioners who think astrologically don't need prompting lists because they already know their etiology and anatomy! Simply apply the thoughts "excessive, impaction, engorgement, tissue growth, massing, and strength" to the zodiac sign (Body Zone) of your patient's natal North Node. Then, consider all the chronic or congenital maladies that might express themselves over time in that manner in that place.

Example: (See Figure 8, page 37, illustrating North Node in Capricorn.) Let us imagine that your patient was born when the North Node was in Capricorn (Body Zone 10). Automatically, then, you know that they might exhibit some tendency toward thickened skin, strong knees (or conversely, gouty knees), and gall stones.

Approach to Treatment

Should symptoms manifest within the body zone of the patient's natal North Node, treatment modalities would include methods to relieve toxic buildup, diffuse fluidic pressure, reduce surplus influx of vital force, and soften.

Please note that sometimes the North Node indicates nothing more than extra strength within that Body Zone. The North Node becomes important only should symptoms suggest this is so.

NIGHT

Stars over snow
   And in the west a planet
Swinging below a star —
   Look for a lovely thing and you will
   find it
It is not far —
   It will never be far.

– Sara Teasdale

Chapter 9

THE PLANETS: HEALTH INFLUENCES

The preceding energetic comparison of Mars (hot, dry, fast) versus Saturn (cold, dry, slow) is easy for beginners to comprehend. Understanding these malefics, alongside the two Lunar Nodes *(Chapters 5-8)*, helps the beginner get started right away. These are the "Big Four" astrological precursors of disease.

What about the other planets? It is best in introductory texts to be as simple as possible when describing planetary action upon the body. For readers eager to put a toe in the water, I've included choice keywords for each planet. More exhaustive discussions on the pathological actions of all planets and both Lunar Nodes are available in my other works. However, you will find plenty of detail here too.

The planets are traditionally known to emit subtle cosmic light of various colors and tones. Planetary vibrational frequencies, both natal and current, influence our health!

Every entity is on certain vibrations. Every dis-ease or disease is creating in the body the opposite or discordant vibrations with the conditions in a body-mind and spirit of the individual. If there are used certain vibrations, there may be seen the response. In some it is necessary for counter-action, in some it is necessary for changes....
– Edgar Cayce (extract from reading), 1861-1912

Planetary Energetics and the Six Tissue States

In *The Practice of Traditional Western Herbalism*, author Matthew Wood brilliantly outlines "six tissue states," attributing them to Dr. Joseph Thurston's "little known tome," *The Philosophy of Physiomedicalism*, 1900. Thurston's work can be seen as further development upon the ancient Greek's four states, well known throughout the literature of traditional astrology and Galenic medicine.

These six tissue states are: hot, cold, dry, moist (traditional Galenic), plus tense, and relaxed (traditional non-Galenic).

A planet's energies, or rather, their impact on the body, can be categorized by two or three of these tissues states each. For instance, Jupiter is "warm and moist." However, I would add two more considerations to the tissue state roster: *fast, slow.* Let me explain.

Normally, heat creates "fast" (stimulating), but not always! There is also a relaxing warmth (think of a hot tub). Energetically, hot and dry are stimulating (speeding up, fast); whereas hot and moist are relaxing, and slowing. (This explains why Mars, a noted hot, dry planet, behaves so very differently when in Water signs.)

Conversely, we think of cold as slowing, as we will shut down and die if left uncovered in frigid temperatures. However, astrologers recognize a form of highly stimulating electric cold in the action of the planet Uranus (think of hot ice). Amongst the planets, Uranus rebels against natural laws.

Herbalist Matthew Wood reminded me that a comparative fast/slow energetic distinction is noted in American Southern and Appalachian folk medicine, in relation to their concept of "fast" and "slow" blood. Sunstroke is considered a result of "fast blood," traditionally recognized in Africa, the Caribbean, and the American South. "Slow blood" corresponds to conditions where the blood grows sluggish, as does the person.

Phyllis D. Light is an Appalachian herbalist of high repute who writes about the Southern and Appalachian traditional system of blood types, in *Southern Folk Medicine*, 2018.

Planets in the 12 Body Zones

Unfortunately, I can't recall the name of the author who wrote that the Body Zone (sign) of a natal planet acts as the reception zone for that planet's energy—similar in manner to a radio's reception of a specific channel. This seems a perfect simile.

According to Hindu tradition, the planets influence us through subtle cosmic light vibrations of various colors. The inestimable Dr. William Davidson explained:

The reason the planets indicate health condition is because flowing into the body are invisible radio-like frequencies, which control and build and maintain all the tissues, and those frequencies are conditioned by the planetary forces in the operation at the first moment of breath, in other words, the cosmos is impressed upon you, the moment you take your first breath.

Because you breathe a cosmic ether as well as air: the scientist doesn't believe that there is any such thing as a cosmic ether. I prefer to believe the people who can see and who have studied it. And so the ether has a sum total of your vibration, as when you take the cap off a camera lens, the surroundings are impressed on the place; so the reason the planets indicate health is because they indicate the frequencies radiating at that moment.

– *Davidson's Medical Lectures*, Dr. William Davidson, edited by Vivia Jayne, 1979, Published by the Astrological Bureau

Each planet influences the Body Zone (sign) it tenants in the birth chart in the manner best described by its temperature (hot / cold / warm); speed (fast, slow); moisture level (dry, moist); and level of tension (tense, relaxed). However, remember this essential rule:

Planetary positions do not always manifest physically; not all planetary positions result in disease!

Planetary influence, if pathological, can manifest physically as various maladies related to the bodily region it tenants. Advanced practitioners know too, that planetary influences can extend or "reflex" to other signs on the season wheel as well. Discussion of planetary reflex to other signs, plus lists of maladies by each planet and Lunar node per sign, is available in *Medical Astrology: A Guide to Planetary Pathology*. There are other authors with similar lists in their books (Nauman, Garrison, Davidson).

Health influences attributed to the two Lunar Nodes through each sign are available in *The Lunar Nodes, Your Key to Excellent Chart Interpretation*, Chapter 8, "The Medical Nodes."

Lists vary, as diseases are endless, and no single author can exhaust them all!

Every planet governs specific diseases and cures. Each planet also governs various glands, hormones, etc. Each planet is assigned a metal, stones, herbs, and various cures both sympathetic and antipathetic. *(See reference books in this book's Bibliography.)*

Yes, this is complex and takes years of training. That being said, it is also true that our *Four Precursors of Disease* offer the healer four immediate keys to diagnosis, treatment, and most importantly, prevention! Although Saturn, Mars and the two Lunar Nodes have their very own preceding chapters, I've included them again here for your convenience, with some additional tips.

Pay attention, first, to Saturn, and next to Mars and the two Lunar Nodes. Remember, in many cases, disease process tends to start with Saturn's placement. This simple method will row your boat. Once you grasp Saturn, Mars, and the Nodes, as previously laid out, then you are ready to advance forward to a complete study of all planets.

Also included in this book are two exhaustively detailed chapters devoted to the distinct medical characteristics of all twelve Sun signs, and again for all twelve Moon signs, so useful to understanding your patient.

Caveat: Planetary influences sometimes produce physical symptoms or maladies within the Body Zone (zodiac sign) tenanted at birth. The word to note is "sometimes." The seeds of any condition may lie dormant, hatching under various stressors including those of cosmic origin. As a lay person, you need not concern yourself with how an astrologer might determine if a planet is "afflicted" because this is a more advanced technique.

Your patient's symptoms should suffice in leading you in the right direction, with stethoscope and horoscope in hand. Additionally, some persons are genetically predisposed to certain conditions as suggested by the planetary position by sign. Others push their own tendencies through deleterious habits.

Remember: Not all planetary positions in the natal chart manifest physically! That being said, Mars, Saturn, and the South and North Lunar Nodes are more likely than the other planets (including the two Lights: Sun and Moon) to do so, especially in genetically predisposed persons, or for those who help along their own negative potentials.

The Planets and Lights

Note: Saturn, Mars, and the Lunar Nodes, while enjoying their own preceding chapters are included here again, with added detail.

SUN (Sol): *The Vital Force, Life Battery, and Light*

The Sun does not necessarily produce palpable heat in the sign tenanted at birth (as does Mars) but, instead, expresses whatever element "he" is tenanting at birth. For instance, when the Sun is in Cancer, the energetic influence is predominantly "cold and moist," despite the Sun being notably "hot and dry." Adhere to Sol's seasonal influence.

The strength and position of Sol in the birth chart indicates the innate quantity and quality of the Vital Force. Think of a battery! Dr. Davidson likened the Sun to electrical voltage, and the Moon to amperage.

Body Associations: The Sun co-rules the heart (with Leo). He governs the brain (with Luna, Mercury, Aries and Taurus). Sol governs the right eye in males and the left eye in females.

Associated Maladies: Sol is associated with stroke, aneurism, heart attack, hypertension, migraines, glaucoma.

Chapter 10 includes a thorough description of medical idiosyncrasies and treatment tips per Sun sign. The Sun sign is another way of saying the sign you were born in.

MOON: *The Moon Distributes the Vital Force*

The natal Moon describes the manner and rate of flow of the vital force, the cycles of circulating fluids and electromagnetic currents. Luna rules the tides as much as she does all manner of monthly biorhythms and fluidic tides, including menses and the blood plasma. She also governs absorption, adaption, and sensitivity. Chapter 11 elucidates Luna's action through each of the twelve signs, in respect to a patient's needs.

Cold and moist (warmer in Fire signs, drier in Earth signs). The Body Zone (sign) that hosts the natal Moon is typically more sensitive, reactive and prone to fluidic extremes (if afflicted, and in predisposed persons). Lunar conditions respond well to tonics, stimulants, astringents, gentle nurturing and drying warmth. However, avoid any drying treatments should the natal Moon be in Fire signs: Aries, Leo, Sagittarius.

Body Associations: Luna co-governs the stomach, breasts, and mucus membranes with the sign Cancer; and the womb with Scorpio. She holds a profound influence over menses and the female hormones (with Venus), especially progesterone. The Moon holds considerable influence over brain function, as does the Sun, Mercury and the signs Aries (upper brain), Taurus (base). She influences the meninges, and the pleural membrane. In concert with Mercury and Gemini, she influences the action of the lungs, and everything "tidal." She rules over the right eye in a female and the left eye in a male.

Associated Maladies: Luna influences the maladies associated with the above mentioned bodily functions and governs over the waters and moisture level of the entire body. Also, "lunacy," (an old medical term). The Moon plays a significant role in brain chemistry related mental illness, as well as mood and eating disorders.

MERCURY: Sense Reception, Nerves

Nervous, fast, generally cold, but warmer in Fire signs, he is a known chameleon who takes on the character of the sign he passes through. The Body Zone (sign) hosting natal Mercury is typically more prone to nervous tension. Mercury conditions respond well to a combination of sedative and nutritive nervines.

Body Associations: Mercury co-governs the peripheral and sensory nerves, hands and fingers (with Gemini) and speech. He greatly influences the speed of the neural synapses.

Associated Maladies: Mercury is implicated in epilepsy (with Uranus and Moon); speech complaints, hearing problems, and all manner of cognitive disorders.

VENUS: *Pain Relieving, Relaxing*

The effect of Venus is magnetic, relaxed, demulcent, sexy, and either pleasantly warm or refreshingly cool as needed (normalizing).

The areas and organs with the Body Zone (sign) tenanted by Venus are prone to muscular laxity (only if afflicted and in predisposed persons). Sometimes these body parts are pretty! Although Venus is less prone to signify chronic issues, she does produce cysts and is associated with sugar problems, venous relaxation, torpor, atonic muscles and of course, venereal issues. Candida and diabetes are her specialties.

Body Associations: Venus co-governs the kidneys and ovaries (with Libra); the veins (with Aquarius); female genitalia (with Scorpio); and rules sugar, estrogen (with the Moon), and copper levels in the body.

Associated Maladies: Diseases of the above organs.

MARS: *Hot, and Dry*

Muscularly energizing, stimulating, tense, and very hot and dry, (hot and wet in Water signs). Excretion, inflammation, and infection. Hyper-function. (Mars slows down and relaxes somewhat when in Water signs Cancer, Pisces. However will still act to inflame the Body Zones ruled by these signs.)

Mars excretes toxins. He acts to both push outward from the periphery, or to penetrate inward from the surface (attack).

The areas and organs within the Body Zone that natal Mars tenants are prone to the above concerns (especially if afflicted and in predisposed persons). Positively, Mars gives energy, athleticism and muscular strength!

Body Associations: Mars co-rules the adrenals (with Aries/Libra), the male genitalia (with Scorpio), testosterone, the muscles, acids, and iron. He *precipitates the gall* (Cornell). Mars governs the left ear with Taurus.

Associated Maladies: Mars governs male virility, accidents, hemorrhage (with Jupiter, Neptune and the Lunar Nodes); bacterial invasion, parasites, bites, wounds, and muscle problems, strains, and some blood diseases.

JUPITER: Growth and Expansion

Protective, fattening, oily. Warm and moist. Diffusive, spreading warmth. The areas and organs within the Body Zone that natal Jupiter tenants are prone to enlargement, fatty deposits, tumors or overgrowth or too large (only if afflicted and in predisposed persons). If positive, this region is protected, strong, nicely padded and functions well. Jupiter is also a great bleeder in association with Mars. He does everything too much! Jupiter's tumors are usually benign, but not always.

Jupiter's speed responds strongly to the element he passes through (Fire, Earth, Air, or Water). He speeds up bodily processes in Air and Fire signs, slows functions when in the Water signs, and goes flat in Earth signs. Positively, the regions within his natal Body Zone (sign) may be large, healthy, strong and protected.

Body Associations: Jupiter co-rules the liver (with Virgo), and the arterial circulation (with Sagittarius). He has a great deal to do with the blood in general. He rules fats.

Associated Maladies: Jupiter is associated with stroke, aneurism and hypertension (with Sun and Mars); obesity, cholesterol issues, organ enlargement, pituitary disorders, diabetes liver problems.

SATURN: Cold, Dry, and Slow

Astringent, mineralizing, and strengthening, Saturn in Water signs either produces trapped water (torpor) or dehydrated tissue states (atrophy). Hypo-function. Restricts circulation and oxygen. The areas and organs within the Body Zone that natal Saturn tenants are prone to the above concerns, plus tumor (especially if afflicted and in predisposed persons).

Positively, Saturn gives strong resistance, longevity and muscular-skeletal strength.

Saturn is famous for restricting excretion and therefore amassing toxins. Lead is his metal, so look for his influence in all cases of lead or heavy metal poisoning. For cancer prevention, consider cleansing, warming and relaxing the organs and tissues within the Body Zone of the patient's natal Saturn. Saturn's conditions respond to releasing warmth and softening. The area of natal Saturn is almost always tense.

Body Associations: Saturn co-rules the bones, ligaments, nails and tendons (with Capricorn) and the teeth (with Taurus). He governs the gall bladder (with Capricorn, Leo, Virgo and Mars). He governs the right ear with Taurus.

Associated Maladies: "Old Father Time" is associated with all the problems of advancing age: stiffening, broken bones, osteoporosis, dry atrophy asthenia, malnutrition, internal and external dryness; constipation, and deafness (with Mercury). He co-influences the nervous system (with Mercury and Uranus). Saturn conducts the aging process.

URANUS: *Electric, Spasmodic, and Cold*

Produces anomalies and extremes. Reverses electrical current and exhibits puzzling symptoms. The areas and organs within the Body Zone that natal Uranus tenants are prone to spasm, electrical issues, extremes, imbalance and difficult-to-diagnose concerns (only if afflicted and in predisposed persons). Symptoms strike suddenly (and may vanish just as fast). Think about electricity. Magnets and electrolytes can work miracles for Uranus' symptoms.

Body Associations: Electricity

Associated Maladies: Uranus is implicated (with Mercury)

in cases of tremor, epilepsy, spasm, et cetera. He throws hormones and other balances off, producing physical and mental extremes. Electromagnetic pollution and poisoning are under the auspices of Uranus and Neptune. EMF-related issues.

NEPTUNE: *Sleepy, Diffusive, and Psychic*

Draining, leaking, and fatigued, drains off the vital force. Associated with viruses, misdiagnosis. Tepid, warm or cool (depending on the sign). Neptune's symptoms are fluidic and dribbling. His issues are often hidden and hard to diagnose. He is similar in action to the South Node, and rules misdiagnoses.

The areas and organs within the Body Zone that natal Neptune tenants are prone to weakness, fatigue, leaking, strange growths, hidden poisons and viruses (only if afflicted and in predisposed persons). Dr. Davidson states that the position of Neptune can indicate the position of a leak in the etheric body.

Neptune leaks prana (vital force)! This planet is strongly associated with some cancers, perhaps through derangement of the electromagnetic field, creating cellular change, or the action of viruses (more research is necessary).

Body Associations: Neptune rules magnetism. Dr. Cornell places the rulership of spinal fluid under Neptune.

Associated Maladies: Neptune indicates our proverbial Achilles heel, that bodily region most open to the astral world, or psychic influence. It is appropriate to investigate all manner of supernatural possibilities with ongoing "undiagnosable" problems of Neptune's indication. He is also associated with secret poisonings.

This mysterious planet is implicated in all manner of weakened mental states, suicidal ideology, visions, fantasy, involuntary clairvoyance and clairaudience, schizophrenia, and severe depression. The personal willpower is absent in these cases.

PLUTO: *Invading, Hideous, and Pathogenic.*

Temperature and emotional extremes (ice cold to explosive, volcanic heat). Radiation poisoning. Plagues. Dr. Davidson says terrible, intense inflammation; researcher Fritz Brunhubner reports fermentation and putrefaction. Positively, Pluto bequeaths remarkable strength, courage and powers of regeneration. Pluto is implicated in organ transplants, blood transfusions, fecal transplants, genetic alteration, Franken-food, plutonium exposure, cadaver transplants, etc.

Body Associations: Exceptionally slow moving Pluto has not yet been observed through the entire circle of signs. To date, this planet has no firmly established body associations, although, hypothetically, he may influence DNA mutation.

Associated Maladies: (Speculative) Lyme disease, AIDS, HIV, Ebola, strep and staph infection, "designer bugs."

SOUTH LUNAR NODE:
Deficient, Weakening, and Draining

Fatiguing, leaking, and sensitizing. Governs genetically inherited issues (maternal). Drains away the vital force. The South Node is not a planet, but it is traditionally included in planetary attributions lists. The areas and organs within the Body Zone that natal South Node tenants are prone to weakness, leaking and deficiency (only if afflicted and in predisposed persons). Yes, the South Node resembles Neptune in action, but also has substantial differences (a discussion for an advanced text).

Body Associations: The South Lunar Node, also known as "The Dragon's Tail," has influence over the anus (shared with Scorpio), and the soles of the feet.

Associated Maladies: The South Node is associated with wasting diseases, fatigue, sepsis, bleeding, leaking, hidden virus, poisoning, gangrene, excess excretions, skin ailments, and addictions (especially to "downers"), suicidal ideologies, depression, psychic disturbances. Blindness, possession, fear, fatigue, prolapse, isolation, deafness, dwarfism, giantism, severe deficiencies, starvation, involuntary psychic opening, coma, miscarriage, ailments of karmic origin, genetically inherited diseases, and cancer. Some maladies are shared with Neptune and also with the North Node.

Look for leaks in the etheric fabric, genetic memory, miasm, past life memory as related to the Body Zone governed by sign of the natal South Node.

NORTH LUNAR NODE:
Excess, Strengthening, and Engorging

Impacting, obstructing, tissue massing, toxic. Governs genetically inherited issues (paternal). The South Node is not a planet, but it is traditionally included in planetary attributions lists. The areas and organs within the Body Zone that natal North Node tenants are prone to strength, impaction, invasion and engorgement. Toxins amass that can cause cancer, but in a manner wholly different than for Saturn.

The North Node indicates a continual pouring in and building up of pressure, with little outlet (think of a boil); whereas Saturn contracts from within. Resultant symptoms can be similar! Medical astrology here can help you determine the energetic cause behind an impaction or tumor.

Body Associations: The "Dragon's Head" is associated with the mouth and throat (shared with Taurus). Also the brain (shared with Aires).

Associated Maladies: North Node is implicated in skin diseases, arthritis, rheumatism, cancer, growths, sclerotic tissue, boils, blocked ducts or arteries, heart attack, brain diseases and pressure, edema, poisoning, dental impactions, throat afflictions, glaucoma, deafness, aneurysm, boils, sepsis, gangrene.

Addictions, (especially to stimulants), possessions, giantism, dwarfism, compulsions, obesity, compulsive eating, cravings, autoimmune issues, epilepsy, mania, and genetically inherited diseases. Some maladies are shared with the South Node, and also with Saturn and Pluto.

Natal Planets Vs. Current Planetary Influence

At birth, the planets, now aka our "natal" planets, are in a mysterious manner, fixed in time and permanently embedded in our physical pattern. These are the planets of the birth chart. But what of the current-time planets?

Following each human birth, the planets obviously continue along on their merry way! The continued movements of the planets are called "transits." On any particular day, month or year, these transiting planets impact the "permanent planetary resonance pattern" that is symbolized by the natal chart. Each planet lends its specified influence. Saturn cools, Mars heats, etc. This presents the healer with two sources of useful knowledge:

1) **The health tendencies of birth, as shown in the natal chart.**

   These are the first thing we assess, and the dominant topic of this book.

2) **The health effects of the current transits upon the patient's birth chart** *(his/her permanent planetary resonance pattern)*.

   This technique is too advanced, for lay readers. However, this book provides some easy rules that all healers should know (**e.g. no surgeries on eclipses**).

For exceptional detail on the physical manifestations of transits, see *Medical Astrology in Action: The Transits of Health.*

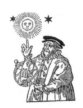

Chapter 10
THE TWELVE SUN SIGNS
A HEALER'S GUIDE

Idiosyncrasies

This chapter details the health idiosyncrasies for the twelve zodiac signs for the use (and amusement) of the attending physician. The expression "Sun sign" refers to the zodiac sign tenanted by the Sun at the day and time you were born.

At the first life breath, we are infused with the character of Solar vital force unique to that specific day of the Solar cycle, within one of twelve zodiac signs. Your patient's birth date is shown in their natal chart by the "degree" and "sign" of the Sun's symbol. This symbol, and its sign also describes the patient's innate quality and quality of vital force.

The natal Sun in the horoscope symbolizes the native's permanent life storage battery of prana. Although the amount we are born with varies with each individual, it is also true that one is free to damage, leak, replenish, or add to their original storage tank.

Important! The idiosyncrasies listed here are sign tendencies, not givens. Many people of all signs go through life in perfect health! Sections are intended for the healer's greater awareness, and not for self-suggestion by those curiously reading about their own sign. Easily suggestible persons should skip this section.

What is a Zodiac Sign?

A zodiac sign is a season of approximately 30 days (varies), pure and simple. The wheel of 12 signs commences each year at the Spring equinox. The Sun-Earth tilt varies daily through the year, providing each day a unique vibrational type of

Solar light. Human beings appear to be infused in some mysterious way with the vibrational resonance of sunlight inherent in their birthday and birth time. The ancients discovered this significant fact, and thousands of brilliant minds have corroborated the truth of this observation.

Regardless of outward appearance, one's innate vital force type, quantity and quality is invariably known by the Sun's position in the birth chart. The physician who knows this fact holds a valuable key to their patient's health.

The Earth-Sun seasonal dance has remained intact since it was first wound up billions of years ago. You may have encountered statements that western astrologers are "using a wrong zodiac because the stars have precessed backwards." True, the stars have precessed, but our zodiac cycle is based on Earth seasons, not stars!

The stars above only approximate the Earth seasons, as markers. Western astrologers do use many specific stars, independently of sign meanings, for other purposes. Our zodiac is not based on star groupings—surprise—but rather upon the yearly dance of the seasons, structured upon a scaffold of two equinoxes and two solstices.

A "Taurus" person is someone born between approximately thirty and sixty days after the spring equinox. In contrast, the sign "Virgo" commences roughly one hundred and fifty days after the yearly spring equinox, and also just thirty days prior to the autumn equinox.

In Western "tropical" astrology, the romantic names of the twelve signs truly refer to twelve seasonal divisions of the Solar cycle. Each thirty degree sign is further subdivided into three periods of approximately ten days each, called "decans."

You can use the 12 tropical signs (seasons) with total confidence! Outwardly, roughly one in three persons will strongly display the traits of their Sun sign, whereas about half the population will moderately do so. Others are more inclined to display the outward traits of their Moon sign, Ascendant sign, or strongest planets.

Despite this variation, all persons possess a life battery, the vital force, and this force permanently infuses and informs their vital force type as given by the birth season or sign (as explained further on).

The following section is primarily for the Sun (birth date) in each of these signs. For illustrations of the physical types, see my book *The Astrological Body Types*. Centuries of empirical observation have documented certain physical traits to the signs.

Caveats: Persons born at sunset and midnight are strangely more apt to outwardly display the traits of their opposite sign! In these cases, pay attention to the Sun sign's Body Zone (sign) as a possible weak spot.

This chapter elucidates the most reliable tips on the treatment for the "natives" of each sign. Because this is a basic text, we have omitted discussion of the Four Elements and Three Modes (each sign belongs to one of each class). Distinctive detail on the quality of each sign's vital force, the Elements and Modes, plus more medical manifestations of both the Sun and Moon through the twelve signs is available in: *Medical Astrology: A Guide to Planetary Pathology*; and *The Astrological Body Types*.

Aries Sun: Medical Tips for Healers

The vital force is strongest in Body Zone 1 (head), manifesting as fast, dry heat in that region. The Aries vital force (prana) is very strong in spurts.

Always give special attention to the brain and eyes. High, sudden fevers are typical. Stroke preventative measures are always a good idea. Physicians and oncologists should be aware that medical radiation directed to the brain of Aries natives may well impact them far more rapidly and powerfully than is typical, or expected. Think twice.

The Aries type needs exercise. As patients, they can be impatient and disinclined to bed rest or appropriate convalescence, but seldom need it, either!

Aries types recover speedily, but can expire speedily too! If they do not expire by accident, Aries and Taurus are the longest-lived signs. The early Spring provides its natives with wondrous vitality!

There is a strong tendency to dehydration, especially of the brain, and towards dry stomach. "Dry eye" is common. The cooling and moistening remedies are often helpful. Peach leaf is a specific for "Aries nausea." Aries runs acid.

The Aries type requires enough cold-pressed oils for good brain function. The adrenal glands are stressed in this sign, so adrenal support is helpful if symptoms present. Aries patients are typically sharp-eyed, cheerfully positive, and alert, muscularly springy, and occasionally irritable. Their dislike of negative thinking works beautifully in the healer's favor!

Aries types are usually attracted to all those things that push their natural heat over the edge: stimulants, chili pepper, caffeine, and the Sun. Then, when overstimulated, they seek something cold and relaxing: booze, or big, icy soft drinks.

Contrary to opinion, it is the Fire signs that are the great drinkers of the zodiac! Curiously, alcohol doesn't appear to damage them as much as it does Water and Earth signs. Those born with Fire-sign Moons share this tendency.

Aries' balancing sign is Libra. Attend to kidney insufficiency, acid/alkaline balance (Aries runs acidic), and hormonal balances (Aries runs toward excess testosterone). Should headache be an issue, check for mineral deposits in the tiny tubules of the kidney, or other kidney issues.

Upset stomachs and nausea are common, especially for Aries Moon. Demulcent herbs and reducing stomach acid is helpful. Peach leaf tea is a specific. Marshmallow and chickweed are also useful.

Tip: The Aries patient born at midnight or sunset may appear more as a Libra!

Aries are prone to "hot-headed" complaints: stroke, fever, mania, hyper-adrenaline, hyperthyroid, ADHD, vertigo, migraine, headaches, meningitis, seizures, accidents, tinnitus, shingles, eye complaints, etc. Fire signs rule Light and respond well to color therapy! Green and blue are the most helpful colors for overheated Aries types.

Weaknesses may lie in the upper intestinal organs and liver-pancreas action (Body Zone 6, Virgo); kidney function and ovarian hormones (Body Zone 7); and excretory/sexual functions (Body Zone 8, Scorpio). As a sign, Aries exhibits a heightened tendency for diabetes, especially when Virgo planets are present in the birthchart.

Taurus Sun: Medical Tips for Healers

Vital force gathers most in the ear-mouth-throat-neck area (Body Zone 2). The strength and endurance of the Taurean vital force is legendary. As children, the Taurus Sun and Moon natives are prone to mucus build-up in these regions and its subsequent consequences. The Moon in Taurus is even more mucus prone in this region. Always attend to the diet and the ear-nose-throat.

Taurus is the longest-lived sign, according to two separate studies. The heaviest babies are born in this sign, and the highest percentage of people in *Who's Who* are Taurus born. What's not to like about being born in mid-May? This is the most magnetic of all signs, full of abundant mid-spring energy.

Taurus rules the mouth; many Taureans are avid foodies,

starting young. Always inquire as to the diet. Taurean types enjoy rich, cheesy, meaty, and sweet foods (as much as possible)—and they like their beer. Most of their problems stem from overeating of inappropriate foods. The liver tends towards torpor in Earth-sign natives, and can grow toxic over time.

Taurus' opposite sign, Scorpio (Body Zone 8), requires their special attention. Taurus is a toxin-retentive sign, ruling the mouth or intake point, whereas Scorpio, governs the colon. There is a significant partnership between Scorpio and Taurus. The mouth and the anus are opposite ends of the digestive track, and thus connected!

Tip: When the Taurus person presents gravel-voice, frequent sore throats, boils, acne, etc., you know it's time to clean the colon! Taurus is prone to all manner of auto-toxic maladies. Taurus natives born at midnight or sunset may more resemble Scorpio.

Taurus is a calm, strong, and magnetic sign. They take well to medical advice, are generally obedient, and can handle convalescence if spoiled in bed with affection and treats.

This sign builds muscle and bone quickly. Even the rare slender Taurus will be strongly-built. Taurus assimilates nutrients well, so bones and wounds mend faster and stronger for them than many other signs.

Regretfully, I cannot remember where I read these things; however, this sign builds habits just as well as muscle mass. Once you get Taurus on a good program, the battle is largely won. Conversely, it may be impossible to break them of cherished bad habits!

Natives of this sign enjoy building projects, gardening, artistic design, cooking, baking, stones, herbs, and plants. These activities are helpful in initiating their healing response.

Taureans respond to beauty in form and sound more than most other signs. This is the veritable sign of "beauty in form."

A diet of visual and musical beauty is very helpful. My definition of beauty: "Harmonies in sound, form, taste, or smell that are helpful and healing to the human mind and body—and for most mammals too!"

Taurus is prone to obesity, food addictions, deafness, dental and jaw complaints, TMJ, neck problems, throat afflictions, tonsillitis, strep throat, vocal polyps, salivary gland obstruction, constipation, boils, abscesses, sepsis, tumor growth, autotoxicity, obstructions, engorgement, impactions, massing of toxins and, especially for Taurus Moon, migraine.

Weakness may be present in kidneys, ovaries, and lumbar (Body Zone 7); genitals, colon, uterus, prostate, bladder, excretory system, nose (Body Zone 8); and hips, thighs, arterial circulation, and lower spinal nerves (Body Zone 9).

Gemini Sun: Medical Tips for Healers

The vital force strongly infuses Body Zone 3: the peripheral nerves, speech centers, bronchial tubes, upper lungs, shoulders, arms, and hands. This sign also governs the capillaries. Continual attention should be paid to strengthen the respiratory organs. Always take a respiratory complaint seriously with this sign, no matter how minor. Gemini is prone to the bronchial complaint that never leaves, slowly exhausting the system, and once weakened, blooming into pneumonia, or even tuberculosis.

The nervous system is overactive in this sign. Natives are highly alert, talkative, high-strung, and fascinated with many things. Unfortunately, Geminis now live in an age where their naturally fast synapses are overloaded with computers, cell phones, and their beloved social media. Gemini is prone to media and phone addiction like none other!

The strain on the nervous system is compounded with snacking on junk, irregular sleep, and poor diets. Nourishing the nervous system and lungs will go a long way to maintain Gemini natives in good form.

Make sure the Gemini patient breathes correctly—this sign governs inspiration, whereas its opposite sign in the yearly wheel, Sagittarius, rules expiration. Gemini, together with Aquarius, governs oxygenation.

Mineral-rich foods, herbs, and roots are useful to ground the jumpy Gemini system. The neurally-exhausted Gemini has usually run themselves down with irregular habits and snacking on junk food. Persons of this sign would be quite healthy if they only took better care of themselves!

Speech and gesture are Gemini functions. Persons born in this month so often evince a hyperactive verbal center in the brain. Learning disabilities are common in childhood. Constant gesticulation is a reliable indication that the horoscope has a strong Gemini component! Gemini governs the coordination of the peripheral nerves, and communication between the two halves of the brain. So often one notes exotropia.

Their opposite sign, Sagittarius, provides Gemini a key to health balance: leg exercise and muscular aerobics. Gemini natives born at midnight or sunset may, in fact, resemble more their opposite sign, Sagittarius.

Slowing down and investing in a program of regular, warm meals in a quiet environment (with the e-devices put away) is in order. The distracted Gemini type person requires someone else to organize a regular schedule for them, as they will rarely do this of their own accord.

As a sign, Gemini is highly prone to asthma, bronchitis, ADHD, nervous exhaustion, ergonomic or repetitive-use complaints of the arms and hands, speech and cognitive disorders insomnia and nervousness. Be alert for gaming, chatting, and phone addiction.

Hidden weakness may be present in colon, bladder,

genitals (Scorpio: Body Zone 8) and skin, bones, knees, and joints (Capricorn: Body Zone 10). It is interesting to note how many persons with asthma or chronic bronchitis (Gemini zone) also suffer rheumatic, arthritic, or skin conditions (Capricorn) or colon problems (Scorpio).

Cancer Sun: Medical Tips for Healers

Body Zone 4. The vital force moves inward to the stomach, breasts, womb, personal memories and receptive feelings.

Natives of Cancer are renowned for their sensitivity on all levels. The defense mechanism works overtime in Cancer; expect all manner of allergies or walling-off mechanisms, from cysts to agoraphobia. This sign strongly influences the pituitary and hypo-thalamus.

Cancerians are extraordinarily sensitive to temperature change and typically run cool—make sure your office is not too cold. The vital force of this sign is notably weak and more compatible with Moon light than sunlight. Avoid prolonged hot tub and sun exposure. Cancereans often prefer night hours.

Cancer, as a sign, is prone to near sightedness and has resistance to physically interacting in a fast manner with the outside world. It is amazing how many Cancerian children are reluctant to bike, swim, or roller-skate. Above all other signs, Cancer needs to feel secure and comfortable. Work to reduce fear (the main emotion of this type). Miasm, family patterns and childhood trauma may play a larger role in apparent health maladies than in most signs.

Cancerian women (and some men) are prone to eating disorders: anorexia, orthorexia, or conversely, food addictions, or compulsive eating. Intervention is sometimes required. Always start with the stomach, but don't neglect the emotions. This sign responds to kindness and affection like none other. Mood control therapy is essential to Cancer's health.

Cancer's opposite sign, Capricorn, provides a useful key: discipline. Also, Capricorn warns the Cancer native to focus on strong bones and mineral assimilation, often weak in this sign. Muscular exercise is important, but sometimes eschewed.

Note: Cancer natives born at midnight or sunset often more closely resemble their opposite sign, Capricorn.

Physical sensitivity is heightened in this sign. Cancerians are acutely sensitive to sound, bright light, Moon phases, fluidic changes, hormones, and temperature. Many wilt under a hot sun and prefer night hours!

This sign is all about personal feelings. Few signs are as responsive to movies and music as is Cancer, and parents of Cancerian children are wise to staunchly shield their children's musical and visual input. Above all, avoid images of horror or terror. For Cancer natives, the mental diet is as essential to health as good food!

Address the lymphatics, as this is a Water sign and governs the thoracic duct. Cancerians are prone to extraordinary hormonal shifts and fluidic retention, especially around the Moon-ruled menses—Cancer is ruled by the Moon!

The memory is remarkable in this sign. It may be productive to address trapped energy patterns from past experience (this life or the last). This sign is noted for family-of-origin issues, unresolved anguish regarding a parent, or abandonment; Bach flower essences work well.

This is one of most musical signs. The right music can heal.

Cancer is also one of the three most fertile signs! Give attention to the breast tissue, and be on the alert for cysts.

Assisting with hormonal regulation and edemic issues is high on the list for members of this sign.

In review, Cancer maladies include: fluidic retention in abdomen, breasts, or brain; overburdened lymphatics; eating disorders and addictions, introversion, emotional memory hangovers, overeating, anorexia, fear, dark moods, fatigue, allergies, immune defense mechanism disorders, pericardium issues, meninges issues, sensitive skin sensitive hearing, temperature swings and sensitivities female hormone extremes, pituitary hormone problems, and breast growth or cyst issues.

Natives of this sign are so often hypersensitive to sound, and should never be expected to convalesce with constant beeping noises or racket about them. A diet of beautiful music is as important as food for members of this spiritual sign. In fact, they are often excellent musicians and singers. If the home environment is pleasant, the Cancerian patient will be vastly happier convalescing at home. These are family people!

Weakness may exhibit in hips, thighs, arterial system, and lower spinal nerves (Sagittarius: Body Zone 9); bones, teeth, knees, structure, skin (Capricorn: Body Zone 10); and circulatory system, veins, and oxygenation of blood (Aquarius: Body Zone 11).

Leo Sun: Medical Tips for Healers

The vital force infuses Body Zone 5: the heart, spinal sheath and thoracic region. The Sun governs Leo and therefore imparts the sign extra vital force.

Leo is the hottest of all signs with heat-related complaints to match. Always be alert for signs of dehydration. Look to the gallbladder—this sign is prone to gall stones and gall malfunction. Leos often exhibit GERD, acid reflux, and other symptoms of what the ancients conceived as "internal heat." Cooling, moistening, and relaxing remedies work quickly to antidote this over-heated sign. Many Leos intuitively know this, resorting to beer and booze. This only dehydrates them further. Leo really needs plenty of pure water!

These natives do best with cooling fruits and salads. It is amazing how often I encounter a Leo strolling about, nursing a carbonated Big Gulp with ice, even in winter. Be on the alert for excessive alcohol consumption.

The heart is governed by Leo (Body Zone 5). Typically, Leo starts life with a strong heart and winds up with high blood pressure, due to lifestyle choices. Leos are very prone to hypertension, stroke, and aortic aneurysm. A flushed-face Leo with red palms should instantly warn you of dangerously building internal heat.

Leo rules the back, in general, but more specifically the spinal sheaths and the thoracic vertebrae. Scoliosis is typical. Leos need to eat to support their spinal sheaths.

I considered this an odd tradition until encountering my first chart of a man with advanced muscular sclerosis (due to disintegration of the spinal sheath). He was a Leo, born with five planets in Leo, a true "stellium." Of course, persons of all Sun signs can get this disease, but in their charts, the signs Leo and Aquarius are typically involved.

Their opposite sign, Aquarius, provides Leo's key to perfect health: balance the venous and arterial circulation. Leo governs the heart, and Aquarius the general circulation—especially the venous. Aquarius also hints at calming and regulating the electrical field (Aquarius rules electricity), and guess what? The Leo-ruled heart is a major electrical generator for the body.

Aquarius also rules the lower legs and ankles. A secret here exists, bequeathed to us from the ancients. If one works with the lower leg and ankle, there is a balancing influence on the heart and also upon the electrical activity throughout the body and heart.

Work to reduce excess heat in the liver and heart. Support the integrity of the spinal sheaths. Attend to spinal subluxations and back problems. Hydrate, hydrate, hydrate! Cool and moisten the body throughout. The heat is often baking down deep in the internal organs—the liver and stomach—and infusing through the heart, spinal cord, arteries, and veins. Reduce caffeine, stimulants, spices, alcohol, and red meat. (Many Leos overdo all three.)

Leos need oxygen, too. Fire without oxygen smolders, and it is precisely this smoldering effect one so often observes. Above all, support heart function.

Weaknesses may reside in gallbladder, bones, joints, and ligaments (Capricorn: Body Zone 10); venous circulation, calves and ankle, electrical issues (Aquarius: Body Zone 11); and lymphatic system, feet (Pisces: Body Zone 12).

Virgo Sun: Medical Tips for Healers

In Virgo, the Solar vital force strongly infuses Body Zone 6: the upper digestive organs including the upper intestines, duodenum, pancreas, liver, appendix, and spleen. Above all, attend to these organs in the Virgo native.

The immune system is governed by Virgo and Pisces. In Virgo natives, the immune system works overtime!

Virgo natives function largely in Beta brain wave mode, and need less sleep than most signs. They like being busily useful. However, they are prone to insomnia, overwork, and subsequent neurological burnout.

A nervously active, yet remarkably sturdy sign, Virgo natives are prone to excess work, anxiousness, and insomnia. Virgo appears to govern the sympathetic nervous system, whereas Pisces (Virgo's opposite sign) influences the para-sympathetic nervous system (Hill). This provides a major key to Virgo health: sleep! Above all else, Virgo needs more sleep, rest, and do-nothing time, seldom getting any of these. Premature graying of the hair is common.

Virgo people are fast-moving and busy, always checking

that cell phone. Over time, nervous exhaustion sets in. One rarely sees a jolly, relaxed Virgo. Attend to nourishing and relaxing the nerves and mind.

One rarely has trouble inducing Virgos to take an interest in their health. Normally, they are already obsessed, with purses full of pills, herbal tinctures, etc. It is wise to discover just what combinations they are using, or if they are overly self-prescribed.

Excess daily amounts of vitamins, minerals, and herbs can confuse the nervous system, sometimes doing more harm than good.

Many Virgo natives opt for no-fat diets, partially due to their sensitive livers. Virgo is prone to diets, dietary extremes, anorexia, and obsessive fitness quests. A great many Virgos elect vegan and vegetarian diets. The digestion is finicky in this sign. Although no rule is absolute, never once have I known a Virgo dinner companion to finish their plate.

Don't force a Virgo child to eat what he or she disdains. It is best they graze upon small, simple meals and do not mix diverse types of fats at one meal.

The liver is slow and fussy in most Virgo natives! Also, the mucous membrane of the intestinal tract runs dry in this sign (as does their skin and hair). Demulcents and emollients are useful.

This sign does poorly with dry roughage, e.g. bran. Soft roughage (bean sprouts, cooked vegetables, and fruit) is preferred. Grains seem helpful to this sign. It is interesting to note that the symbol for this sign is a maiden holding a sprig of grain! Raw foods seem to irritate the bowel in this sign.

The Virgo type often suffers from malnourishment or self-starvation. They eat, but often not enough calories to nourish themselves fully, especially in their older years.

As a sign, Virgo is prone to diverticulitis, pancreatitis, Crohn's, colitis, liver and gallbladder problems, and diabetes. Virgo co-rules the pancreas and Islets of Langerhans (with Jupiter). In fact, diabetes is a famous "Virgo" disease, also prevalent in Libra. Sugar is governed by Venus, so this planet must also be afflicted in the birth chart for diabetes to occur. Venus, Saturn, and either Lunar Node in Virgo all say "watch that blood sugar!" Attend to blood sugar levels and the health of the upper digestive tract.

The current trend in food allergy testing is relevant for Virgo natives. Virgo is a tough sign with a strong immune system. Immune response is impressive, and Virgos can be prone to autoimmune issues. This sign works overtime defending the body from intrusion. (Virgo and Pisces are said to govern the immune system.) It is noticed that Virgo people both heal wounds and convalesce quickly, whereas their opposite sign Pisces is slow! Generally speaking, a flu or cold will last half as long for Virgo as for Pisces.

Similar to Leo, Virgo builds internal heat. Both signs (Virgo and Leo) have much to do with gallbladder malfunction, as does Capricorn.

Natives of this sign are prone to lipid deficiency, often presenting as dandruff and dry skin. The premature gray hair common to this sign is possibly indicative of nutritional deficiency.

Virgos are enthusiastic and obedient patients who typically opt for the natural approach, if given that option. Many are excellent lay herbalists themselves! Virgos incline to service, administrative, and medical professions.

Weakness may exhibit in head, eyes, brain (Aries: Body Zone 1); lymphatic system, feet, sleep disorders (Pisces: Body Zone 12); circulation, ankles (Aquarius: Body Zone 11). However, their digestive organs are paramount!

Libra Sun: Medical Tips for Healers

The vital force strongly infuses Body Zone 7: the kidney, ovaries and lumbar region. Libra, the sign of the scales, governs balances. Salt balances, electrolyte balances, fluidic and hormonal balances, and acid/alkaline balance are under the province of this sign. Typically, Libras appear relaxed and in good health. However, they are seldom attentive to health and are often "sugarholics." Diabetes is as prominent for Libra as it is for Virgo and Aries.

Beautiful hair, skin, and melodious voices attest to the Libran affinity with Venus, the planetary ruler of estrogen and copper. Attend to any sugar or wine habits early, and support the kidney function. Should acne present, look to kidney filtration and hormonal imbalance. Venus-ruled Libras either have lovely skin or acne.

Clue: For natives of Libra, a disturbed kidney filtration outlets onto the face. Scorpio is acne-prone too, but for quite different reasons. Medical astrology readily discerns the difference. Dr. Davidson described how headaches are so often caused by poor kidney filtration, typical of Saturn's placement in Libra. Libra rules the kidneys, and its polar opposite sign, Aries, rules the brain.

Libra natives dislike diets and compulsory exercise. Unless a healthy dose of Fire signs exists in their horoscope, Libra hates to move. Natives of this sign have the curious faculty of being able to live off junk food for years and be none the worse for it. Eventually, though, after age fifty, the sugar, alcohol, cigarettes, romances, etc., take their toll. Diabetes runs high in this sign.

The ovaries are governed by Libra (shared with Venus), so it's wise to keep an eye on ovarian health. Hormonal and adrenal balance is essential. The adrenals are governed by the Libra-Aries polarity and the planet Mars.

Libra natives are strongly influenced by partners and spouses on all levels. This is the sign governing marriage, although this instinct just as easily manifests as compulsive partnering. A happy marriage makes a happy Libra! If health is awry, it is wise to discover what is going on with the current relationship or partner. If the partner is ill, the health status of a Libra native suffers too.

Libras do well to seek balance in all things: diet, exercise, sex, rest, and work. Libra signifies a need to balance mental, social, and physical activities. Avoid extremes! A Libra's opposite sign, Aries, provides a valuable key to health, i.e., aerobic exercise. Libra prefers partnering, even in exercise (for example, tennis). At least, find them a walking partner.

Weaknesses may lie in Body Zone 12: the lymphatic filtration (sluggish), and the feet; Body Zone 1 (head, brain, eyes, adrenal action), and Body Zone 2: the thyroid, ear-nose-throat region. However, the kidneys are the main thing!

Scorpio Sun: Medical Tips for Healers

The vital force strongly infuses Body Zone 8: the colon, bladder, genitals, general excretory system, and curiously, the nose! The vital force is supremely powerful in this sign and capable of regenerating the body, even from the most grievous of complaints. Never assume a "mortal" illness is mortal for a native of Scorpio. This is the sign of the proverbial "cat with nine lives," and the native so often gets their chance to prove it, too!

Scorpio natives are prone to acne, profuse sweats, and other indications of active excretions. I've encountered more than one Scorpio-born who must rush to the hospital with dangerous nose-bleeds. However, it is plausible that Scorpios might suffer less from cancer than signs that hoard toxins! The

Scorpio's excretory system works overtime, and your problem as a healer becomes one of how to assist in the removal of excess toxins flowing liberally from the lymphatics, blood, kidneys, nose, uterus, and colon.

Always support excretion and blood filtration for Scorpio natives. In the old times, Scorpio maladies were caused by "dirty blood." Scorpio blood runs acid, so alkaline diets are best. Pure water is necessary, as Scorpio is a "fixed" Water sign, suggesting stagnant water. Scorpio does well with lymphatic-clearing herbs. Poke root tincture is a good contender. Red Root, Burdock, and beets are excellent. These and other alterative "blood clearing" herbs are excellent choices, as Scorpio is prone to excess hormones in the bloodstream, morbid acne, boils, foul smelling sweat, etc.

Scorpios enjoy and indulge in intense food flavors: kumquats, kimchi, fermented foods, designer chocolates, liqueurs, chili peppers, garlic, etc. They are also prone to excessive tobacco, alcohol, and opiate consumption. Scorpios enjoy decadent deserts as much as do the Taureans!

Other common conditions encountered are: nasal infections, nose bleeds, bladder infections, bladder cancer, diarrhea, endometriosis, vaginal candida, bacterial overgrowth in the colon, prostate issues, fungus, hemorrhoids, hernia, appendicitis, colitis, prolapsed uterus, Crohn's disease, STDs, herpes, and all manner of genital / sexual issues.

Take heed—this sign is uniquely prone to bacterial imbalance, fungal infection, parasitical infestation of all kinds, and nasal and bladder infection. It is unclear why natives of this sign are prone to parasitical symbiotic conditions.

As perhaps the most courageous sign, Scorpios are so often attracted to dangerous occupations with attendant risk of contamination from body fluids, poisons, mold, bacteria, foul water, chemicals, or vermin (recall that renowned Scorpio native, chemist Madame Curie). When encountering a Scorpio with a sticky problem, a little detective work on your part into their daily work and home environment is typically rewarding.

Scorpios almost universally love dogs, which often share their beds.

Their sex life is sometimes experimental or extreme. Curiously, one study showed that more celibate monks and nuns are born in Scorpio than any other sign. Scorpios I've interviewed are, indeed, celibate for long years, alternating with periods of experimental sexual extremes. (Scorpios, please take no offense, as no single astrological observation is true for all.)

Scorpio's opposite sign, Taurus, provides a key to good health: good, natural food. (Taurus rules the mouth.) What goes in must come out. Scorpio rules the tail end of that cycle! The thyroid is sensitive in both signs, and often hypofunctioning.

Because Scorpio rules the nose, it may well be that Scorpios respond strongly to aromatherapy! All manner of nasal issues and hemorrhages are common.

Scorpio has the greatest powers of self-suggestion and hypnosis of all signs, well able to reverse the course of dire diagnosis, if only you tell them they might do so. These natives are also curious about all things medical, and notoriously fearless. You can be very direct with them. I recall my Scorpio father insisting on having his root canal procedure performed without anesthesia because he "found pain interesting." Natives of this amazing sign are the greatest healers of the zodiac, and make wonderful surgeons!

Visualization techniques are also super-effective for this sign. Once, a semi-literate, older female truck driver came to a medical astrologer after a diagnosis of certain death within three months from a cancer nobody survives. "I am not a statistic," she protested.

The medical astrologer replied, "All right; then, try the classic visualization of white knights (white blood cells) attacking the cancer." She did so, and her "incurable" cancer vanished straight away without a trace, much to the astonishment of her physicians. This is all par for the course for Scorpio natives. There the Scorpio "victim" sits, years later in perfect health, having survived one or more mortal ailments! If your patient is a Scorpio, remember this!

Scorpio health is bountiful if the healer attends to the toxic clearance of the blood, lymphatics, kidneys, bacterial balance of the colon, and colon function. Weaknesses may include the upper lungs and bronchial tubes (Body Zone 3: Gemini); thyroid, throat, ears (Body Zone 2: Taurus); and brain, eyes (Body Zone 1: Aries). However, their own bodily regions are paramount (Body Zone 8).

Sagittarius Sun: Medical Tips for Healers

The vital force strongly infuses Body Zone 9: the central nervous system, arteries, lower spinal nerves, hips, thighs, and voluntary muscles.

This is a toe-tapping, restless, and athletic sign, generally cheering and enlivening to those about them. So many of their problems stem from insufficient free movement and musculo-skeletal issues. Sciatica is common. This sign needs to run, walk, and play ball! Should Sagittarians be sedentary, their "muscular fire" will migrate into the nerves, creating restlessness, neuroses, addictions, insomnia, and mental problems.

This sign is prone to religious mania, ADHD, hysteria, panic attack, spinal cord diseases, tremor, epilepsy, schizo-phrenia, bi-polar disorder, and self-medication. Few signs are more prone to hyperthyroid and Grave's disease. Sedative herbs work well with this sign.

This sign governs the arterial system and is prone to hypertension and strokes. Always be alert to this tendency in the type, because if it occurs, it is serious. Fire energy can go wild in this "mutable" Fire sign. Mutable means moving, transitioning between states. Think of wildfire.

Sagittarius natives typically require a high level of excitement and motion. This sign binges, often going days without proper sleep, then crashing. Many Sagittarius natives enjoy the thrill of hurtling through space: driving fast, flying, skate boards, motorcycling, and all manner of wild adventure. More often than not, they eat catch-as-catch-can, and suffer from bouts of insomnia.

Assist the Sagittarius patient with vigorous exercise programs and safe adventures balanced by good sleep. Rolfing, osteopathy, yoga, Pilates, t'ai chi and all kinds of "body work" are compatible. Foolish mishaps and stupid deaths are not uncommon! Sagittarius are often eager to try sky diving and other extreme sports, with little consideration of personal danger. It's a good thing they are so lucky.

Be alert for mental extremes and flights of idealism. Sagittarius' opposite sign, Gemini, provides a healing key: live in the here-and-now and avoid being carried off by abstract thoughts at the expense of everyday life. Play without meaning. Balance muscular activity with mental activity and study. In reflex to this same sign, the lungs and bronchial tree may require extra care. Never allow a chest complaint to take hold! Many smoke; no help there.

Unfortunately, most hyperactive Sagittarians adore caffeine. In extreme cases, they seek to further amp themselves up with cocaine or other uppers, relaxing afterward with alcohol. This pattern, seen too often, will burn them out early. Many Sagittarius males expend their life-candle in youthful escapades.

The hips and thighs need special attention, as does the spine. The season of Sagittarius seems to stimulate the spinal nerves, as also does the Moon when she passes through this sign once monthly. Foods and herbs that nourish the spinal nerves and spinal sheath are well worth the investment for natives of this sign. The hips need to be kept strong, and musculoskeletal imbalances ironed out as early as possible. This sign is prone to femur injury and uneven leg growth.

A typical Sagittarius native is happiest playing aerobic, large muscle sports: running, throwing, tennis, baseball, riding horses, archery, and bicycling. Typically, they love dogs as much as does their neighboring sign, Scorpio. Many great equestrians are natives of this sign.

This type sometimes has trouble in school, being far too kinetic for the sit-down classroom. Learning disabilities may be diagnosed and the child drugged, when all they needed was vigorous exercise. Suppressing Fire sign energy with drugs will lead to serious problems down the line.

Although buoyant and cheerful, Sagittarius seems prone to chronic ailments throughout later life, but equally so, rising victorious over them! This is puzzling, but so often the case.

Support the muscles, spinal nerves and sheaths, spinal column, hips and thighs, and thyroid. Focus, calm, and settle the mind. Keep happy the bronchial tubes, lungs stomach. Make sure the diet and sleep life are in order. Inquire as to beverage type and intake.

Weakness may be found in the stomach or breast (Body Zone 4); respiratory and nervous systems (Body Zone 3); and the thyroid, and ear-nose-throat (Body Zone 2). However, their own bodily regions are paramount to health maintenance (Body Zone 9).

Capricorn Sun: Medical Tips for Healers

The vital force strongly infuses Body Zone 10: the knees. The Sun in this sign also profoundly influences the skeletal structure, bones, skin, nails, and cuticles (positive or negative). This season of birth has a drying, hardening influence. Nota bly delicate as infants, they gradually strengthen, and when old, according to Cornell, "...will not die without a push!" I have corroborated his observations.

Consider granite. Now, visualize how granite absorbs sunlight: slowly. A cold granite boulder will gradually absorb the Sun's warmth and yet retain the heat a long time. This precisely describes the life cycle of typical Capricorns. Often, they are surprisingly strong and their endurance is legendary. While not fast starters, they can be counted on to survive famines and long mountain treks.

Liver function is notoriously slow in this sign. Because the gallbladder is co-ruled by Capricorn (with Leo, Saturn, and Mars), gallstones are common. Capricorn is a careful eater, often grazing throughout the day on a rigidly restricted diet of specific foods.

Typically, they do not receive enough calories or fats. The diet may lack variety, and malnutrition quietly ensues. Look for symptoms of scurvy—yes! Suspect that vitamin, mineral, and/or protein deficiencies may loom behind complaints.

Capricorns love grains and frequently prefer a vegetarian diet. However, this sign assimilates calories well, and factually, can thrive on low food intake for years! This is the sign of the monk who lives on groats. This is a good strategy for babies born at winter's onset!

Brittle nails, receding gums and cracked cuticles are typical to the type. With few exceptions, persons of this sign suffer skin, nail, or cuticle issues. Moles, warts, dry skin, dandruff, premature graying, eczema, psoriasis, skin cancers, nail fungus, chipped nails, dry nails, etc., are common. Normal skin protections seem lacking, and/or the lipid metabolism fails to supply the outer surface.

The Capricorn type is well advised to avoid strong sun.

There are two opposite physical types. The Saturnian type is quite lean, even emaciated, with prominent bones, and yet quite strong. The Earth-sign Capricorn type is thickly built with a massive, tough body of hard muscle and hard fat. In fact, many of the great heavyweight boxers were born with their Suns in this sign.

Temperature is hard to understand in this sign. Capricorn natives appear cold and often feel cold. However, due to internal dehydration, heat seems to bake down in the system. The mucous membrane is often too dry and needs moistening. This can produce various digestive disorders and nausea usually targeting the stomach, liver, gallbladder, and sometimes the intestine.

Traditionally, chemical medicines may be vomited up. Laxatives are also less than effective, especially when the Moon transits through this sign! Natives of this sign have sensitive, dry stomachs and deficient digestive acids. Comforting the mucus membrane of the stomach is key.

Rheumatism, arthritis, as well as ligament, tendon, and joint issues are common. Sometimes this is due to simple dehydration, so typical of this sign. However, Capricorn natives are prone to insufficient joint lubrication, poor lipid distribution, and toxic liver. These issues can contribute to dry ligaments and tendons and dried out, inflamed joints.

The memory suffers in this sign, especially after a lifetime of brain dehydration or insufficient fats. Alzheimer's and dementia are common. Support memory!

In sum, always attend to your Capricorn patient's joints, skin, fat digestion, hydration, and gallbladder function.

As a sign, Capricorn is highly prone to uterine fibroids. For years, I noted that, with few exceptions, every female client born with her natal Moon in Capricorn had undergone a hysterectomy! It is obvious that early attention to the uterus is essential for females with this Sun or Moon sign (especially the Moon sign).

Restrained, tense emotions make for brittle problems! The key to balanced health for Capricorn is suggested by its opposite sign, Cancer. Attend to the stomach absorption and mucous membrane. Encourage Capricorn to experience emotional sensitivity, relax, be receptive, and let go of control.

Music therapy is very effective. Encourage them to learn to express affection with plants or pets, or perhaps take a watercolor class. (Capricorn is the great graphic artist, whereas its opposite sign Cancer is the poetic expressionist.)

Capricorns enjoy useful exercise: building, baking, farming, or gardening projects. They prefer digging and hammering to fast aerobics. Capricorn natives are surprisingly tough physically, despite appearances.

Tip: Capricorn patients take well to disciplined health and diet regimens.

Warning: As a rule, Capricorns are modest and dignified. They dislike penetration, shots, undressing for strangers, etc. They react badly to surprises. Always carefully explain everything you are doing—before you do it!

Weaknesses may reside in Body Zone 5 (heart / gallbladder); Body Zone 3 (bronchial tubes, nerves, and lungs); Body Zone 4 (stomach, breast, uterus, mucus membrane, gums, elbow). However, their own bodily regions are of paramount interest in the maintenance of good health (Body Zone 10).

Aquarius Sun: Medical Tips for Healers

The Aquarius vital force strongly infuses Body Zone 11: the calves, ankles, and the little known electrical system of the body. Mid-winter is not an optimum season for birth. Aquarian natives are prone to all manner of "cold" complaints, but with a twist different from neighboring winter signs. For starters, Aquarius governs the little-understood electrical system of the body. Spasm, cramps, and all manner of odd neurological disturbances are associated with this sign, famous for maladies "impossible to diagnose."

Oxygenation of the blood is ruled by Aquarius and Gemini. Strangely, Aquarians reliably suffer sub-oxygenation and prefer sleeping with a window open.

Aquarius governs the general circulation of the blood, most especially the venous circulation (with Venus). Poor circulation, cold extremities, and low blood pressure are typical complaints. The lymphatic system of the brain may require assistance. See Matthew Wood's *Earthwise Herbal Repertory*.

The heart muscle is all too commonly weak in this sign, as is the vital force. If you have an Aquarian patient, be alert for bouts of exceptionally low blood pressure and / or anemia that should never be ignored. Extremities will run cold, and they will complain of fatigue or dizziness.

This sign holds precedence over "the quality of the blood," and a significant percentage of Aquarius Sun and Moon natives exhibit anemia at some point in their lives. Always consider the integrity of the blood cells in your Aquarian Sun and Moon patients.

Depression is another concern, so common to the sign. This malady is nearly invariable for Aquarians born at night, and near the new Moon, signifying a total lack of light! Replacement light therapy is in order for winter-born depression sufferers. Loneliness is common to Aquarius, a personality type few understand. Many Aquarian men, in particular, are isolated, and Aquarians of both sexes often dine alone, or are somehow ostracized from their family of origin.

To reiterate from the preceding, the heart muscle is often weak in this sign, requiring strengthening. Look to see if there is fluidic puffiness about the ankles. Strengthen the heart and half your battle is won.

Another curiosity about this sign is the poor absorption of vitamins and sometimes minerals, too. All things ruled by the Sun seem at a loss: Vitamins A, E, D, magnesium, and iodine. Aquarians crave salt, the mineral that conducts electricity!

This sign co-governs the spinal nerves. Mineral-rich herbs and foods that support and strengthen the nervous system are a significant help to Aquarian patients.

Aquarius is the most sensitive of all signs to barometric changes (Davidson) and EMF fields. It is wise to inquire as to computer, media, and cellphone habits. EMF fatigue is a serious reality, so often passed over. More than most signs, Aquarians benefit from e-vacations, and forest bathing (walking or sitting in forests). Aquarians require fresh air and complete liberty. Typically, they eschew a nine-to-five regime, preferring freelance.

The key to Aquarian health: Oxygen, light, vitamins, circulatory stimulation, blood quality support, iron, heart strengthening, mental upliftment, warmth, and neural nourishment. Warm the body and mind.

Aquarius' opposite sign, Leo, provides the clues to balancing the Aquarian tendencies. The Aquarian native must build a strong heart and vital force, both being natural to Leo. In the Renaissance, a nugget of gold, or bag with three Solar herbs worn over the heart was helpful, and still is! However, I've discovered that one, three, or five large pieces of blue turquoise worn directly over the heart work wonders for Aquarian heart fatigue.

Many Aquarians do well to eat plenty of blood-building red, black and purple foods; e.g. beets, raisins, and seaweed. Sesame seeds help build the integrity of the blood cells and may be useful for these natives (and for Pisces too!).

Aquarians are frequently of above-average intellect. Many are true geniuses in their accomplished field. Aquarian types overindulge in books, science, fascinating mental hobbies, computer use. The imagination is highly active, and fertile. These are your idea people, so prone to mental extremes.

Intellectual activities should be balanced with opposite-sign Leo type activities, e.g. playing with pets, human affection, sports, hiking, dancing, and sense-involvement in present time such as cooking, et cetera.

Bizarre symptoms of possibly electrical origin sometimes require inventive solutions. Consider magnet therapy, charged water, copper water, et cetera. The herbs useful for Aquarius circulatory, heart and blood issues are Rosemary, Sage, Nettles, Yarrow, Hawthorne, and Dulce.

Weaknesses may exhibit in upper digestive organs (Body Zone 6); heart, back, spinal structure (Body Zone 5); and stomach, breasts, uterus, and motherly instincts (Body Zone 4). However, their own bodily regions are of paramount interest for health maintenance (Body Zone 11).

Warning: Aquarius Sun and Moon patients are known to manifest unexpected and extreme reactions to medications and homeopathy. Always test carefully before whole-dosing these patients.

Pisces Sun: Medical Tips for Healers

The vital force strongly infuses Body Zone 12: the feet. The Sun in this sign also strongly influences the lymphatic system, the parasympathetic nerves and the psyche. The last sign of the seasonal cycle is also the sleepiest. "Excessive" sleep is appropriate and natural for natives of this sign.

Pisces is the primary governor of the lymphatic system. One frequently notes a waterlogged cellular matrix and overburdened lymphatic system.

For your Pisces patients, you might consider warming and assisting the lymphatics. Also, work directly through the feet (foot reflexology, massage, oils, etc.). The vital force is perhaps the lowest of all signs, Cancer being another candidate for innately weak vital force.

Pisces seasonal energy is fog-like, diffusively meandering and porous. Never allow flu to take hold, and if ill, allow a long conva-lescence. Do all you can to build up the vital force in Pisces natives, young and old!

Pisces rules "the whole," and is a sign said to contain all signs within it. This is also the season closest to the astral world or, as one might say, "the other side." Therefore, it makes sense why these patients respond best to holistic, whole body, and body-spirit approaches including meditation, prayer, yoga, dancing, ta'i chi, and foot reflexology. Decocted herbs work very well. Herbal treatments, soups, broths, and seaweeds are made for natives of this season!

Pisces natives are more responsive to the unseen world than to this present Earth plane. All manner of vibrational remedies work well for them: homeopathy, music therapy, hypnosis, and Bach flower essences. This is a psychically absorbative sign that requires plenty of diffusion time. Nine-to-five jobs, high-pressure, or noise, speedily exhaust them. Knowledge of psychic self-defense is a must.

All too often, a Pisces patient ails because their parent is dying, or a friend is burdening them with their problems... or maybe the house has a ghost! Your influence as their healer is powerful here, so attend to your vocal tone, choice of office music and what you say. Positive suggestions will go far! Pisces is one of the most musically responsive signs, so it is wise to inquire as to their musical diet.

To understand a sick Pisces, inquire as to their social milieu, work, home, and unseen influences. And, are they getting any alone time to just hang loose? Their vital force is extremely porous. For health, Pisces require more diffusion time than any other sign. Tips for protecting psychic Pisceans from "family DNA resonance problems" are described in *Astrology & Your Vital Force.*

However, for perfect health, we must always balance with Pisces' opposite sign, Virgo; attend to good nutrition, physical fitness, and useful work. Also, attend to the upper digestive organs: liver, spleen, pancreas, duodenum, upper intestine, and cecum. Although Virgo-ruled, these organs may be hypo functioning in Pisces patients. In fact, the cecum, though well outside of Body Zone 12, is considered under the province of Pisces.

Pisces types are prone to hypoglycemia, whereas Virgo types are prone to hyperglycemia and diabetes! Pisceans require spleen support, often exhibiting low white blood cell counts. The weak vital force of this sign doesn't easily throw off viruses and bacteria. The Pisces immune system needs all the help it can get! Sesame seeds help build the integrity of the blood cells and may be useful for these natives.

Pisces runs cold and moist. In some types, the body collects water, and brain function appears waterlogged. Warming stimulants are excellent. Another Pisces type is graceful and fluid.

These natives strongly respond to sympathy and hypnotic suggestion. Healers, be attentive to what you say, how you say it, and your vocal tone. Patient-physician harmony is of utmost importance for natives of this sign. *(See Chapter 14, "Doctor-Patient Relations.")* Neither should a fatigued physician attend to a Pisces patient; they can drain you (being natural prana vortexes), and you will further drain them.

They suffer delicacy as infants and throughout life, often lacking stamina or strength. Pisceans also often assimilate proteins poorly. Building bodily strength and confidence is of supreme importance.

FYI: Hyper-flexibility and slippery ligaments are common to this birth season.

Pisces natives may have slower blood-clearance than others, and often cannot tolerate alcohol or chemical medicines. They can be prone to boils, purple blotches, carbuncles, and wet rashes. As with Aquarius and Gemini natives, low-dose them first and observe responses. Should the Pisces-born abuse their bodies with drugs and alcohol, they seldom last long. There are many famous examples of this in the rock band world!

Pure water and the alterative "blood clearing" herbs are most helpful to natives of this sign. Some lymphatic-assisting herbs for consideration are Dandelion, Burdock, Red Clover, Red Root and Poke Root, Cleavers and Blue Violet. Purple blotches and damp boils are classic to those Pisces who evince their birth season's trait of slow lymphatic and blood clearance.

Similar to Aquarius, Pisces also needs to attend to, and build, the quality of the blood. Beets are the color of Pisces on the color wheel and an excellent choice for this sign.

This sign is famous for lung delicacy, and prone to chronic lung complaints including pneumonia, emphysema and TB. Pisces lungs tend to trap moisture and run cold (unless opposite chart tendencies reverse this—for example, Mars in Gemini— this would instead create hot, dry lung).

Remember, this is the "foot sign!" Keep the feet happy, and look to the feet for mysterious problems higher up in the skeletal chain.

So often, Pisces patients are hypersensitive to sound and, like Cancer, should never be expected to convalesce with constant beeping noises or racket about them. A diet of beautiful music is as important as food for members of this spiritual sign.

There is a tradition that Pisces governs "the coordination of the glands." It is so true that many Pisces-born individuals display signs of glandular excess, or deficiency.

Wholistic processes that are, as yet, little understood may be considered as largely ruled by this sign. These would include the interstitial fluid matrix and glandular coordination. Pre-empt the cognitive decline common to this sign by assisting the lymphatic system of the brain and the smooth functioning of the choroid process. With Pisces, its all about the lymphatics!

The parasympathetic nervous system is clearly most active in the natives of this sign! In studies of narcolepsy, one so often notes many planets in the polarity of the sympathetic-parasympathetic nervous system: Virgo and Pisces.

The sentimental memory is unmatched in this sign! The classic Pisces doesn't easily recover from abandonment or a broken heart, and may loose their will to go on. Homeopathic, or spiritual assistance may need to intervene. A little kindness goes a long way with natives of this most sensitive of signs.

Weaknesses may exhibit in Zone 5 (Leo, the heart); Zone 6 (upper organs of digestion, immune system–low); and Zone 7 (Libra, the kidneys, fluidic balances, and ovaries). However, their own bodily regions are of foremost importance towards the maintenance of their good health (Body Zone 12).

Chapter 11

THE MOON SIGNS
KNOW YOUR PATIENT'S NEEDS

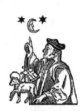

The Moon is so essential to health that I've devoted several chapters to her medical implications in previous works. Let's keep it simple here. Our theme will be "emotional needs," with some critical physical needs tossed in.

If one celestial body describes our needs, it's the Moon. If you want to know your patient's "need type," you must know their Moon sign. This is easy to do, but sometimes requires an accurately timed birth chart because the Moon changes signs approximately every two and a half days. Understanding the emotional requirements of your patient is invaluable knowledge for any healer! In fact, it's a life saver.

Although the natal Sun's sign indicates the storage battery of vital force, the Moon sign indicates its manner and rate of flow! Dr. Davidson likened the Sun to electrical voltage and the Moon to amperage.

The natal Sun indicates the quality and quantity of power, or voltage (of the vital force). The rate, rhythm, monthly perturbations and distribution of the vital force current is governed by the natal Moon. (This tradition was well preserved for us by Dr. William Davidson; *see Bibliography.*) Further description of the Moon governed "rate of flow" by zodiac sign is provided in my book *Medical Astrology: A Guide to Planetary Pathology,* Chapter 5.

Important! The idiosyncrasies listed here are sign tendencies, not givens. Many people of all signs go through life in perfect health! Sections are intended for the healer's greater awareness, and not for self-suggestion by those curiously reading about their own sign. Easily suggestible persons should skip this section.

Aries Moon: Independence, Direct Experience, Doing

Natives of the Aries Moon detest convalescing as much as they do dependency. They'll strive to be active as soon as possible. Aries Moon people crave excitement, stimulation, action, and fun. They are emotionally independent and will probably not follow your directions or regime, (typically, the spouse dragged them to your office in the first place.) The Aries Moon patient requires more hydration to the brain, eyes, stomach than most other signs do, and the mucus membrane may tend to dry inflammation.

This Moon sign is noted for fast, high fevers that strike unexpectedly, and can endanger life! If so, consider cooling and hydrating the brain, and pulling energy to the feet.

Typically, they love sunlight, early morning activities, singing and emotionally charged, rhythmic music (gospel, bluegrass, etc.). Stimulating music and rhythm is healing to them (as long as the chords are harmonious). Disharmonious chords and cacophony do not assist healing. I mention this because some young patients with this Moon sign may prefer agitating racket for its *adrenalizing* impact.

Creativity of all kinds will greatly uplift them, as will laughter. Tell them they can get well and they probably will!

Because Aries Moon natives crave stimulation, the healer must assess if they are imbibing excessive caffeine or energy drinks. Conversely, they so often relax at day's end with alcohol. Be on the alert for brain dehydration.

Taurus Moon: Sense Comfort, Good Food, Beauty.

The Taurus Moon patient loves touch, sense pleasure, good food and smells, and melodic music. They are greatly benefited from beautiful forms about them, so the architecture of the healing environment really does impact them, as does decor. They respond well to physical affection. Pets (to pet!) are a grand idea; plants, gardening, being in a garden—all good.

Physicians should be alert for secret food habits that are contributing to the problem (the nightly ice cream sundae). Taurus rules the larynx and vocal chords, and responds well to therapeutic chants or singing. Building, cooking, drawing, and designing are all up lifting. May require stimulation and excretory assistance.

Be alert for constipation, boils. It is amazing how often you will encounter the Taurus Moon child with ear infections, excess ear wax, tonsillitis, etc. Mucous appears to build readily in their ear-nose-throat region, and dairy is often the culprit.

This sign governs the mouth! More than any other sign, the Taurus Moon craves their favorite comfort foods, and has a taste for rich, sweet and fatty treats. Natural gourmands, they are happiest when well fed. Obviously, this trait can work for or against the doctor!

Gemini Moon: Connection, Communication

The Gemini Moon person needs someone to talk to! These patients enjoy fun and games, puzzles, light reading, diversion, communication, mental entertainment, visitors, surprises, conversation, and most of all, the phone. Gemini Moon natives require more support to the nerves than do most other Moon signs. They perk up with personal coordination exercises, musical instruments, doing things with the hands (carving, drumming, piano, juggling, etc.).

They often smoke cigarettes "...to do something with my hands." Traditionally, this sign reacts strangely to chemical medicines. Although EMF-exposure attenuates their sensitive nerves, it may be difficult to pry them off their devices. Their own health is not as high a priority to them as staying connected. Give attention to the respiratory organs and nerves. Weak, damp lungs, nervous stomach and insomnia are common complaints.

If the Gemini Sun or Moon patient will implement an EMF-free convalescence, half your battle is won. Good luck!

Cancer Moon: Security, Family

The Cancer Moon patient needs family, mom, security, comfort food, tenderness, reassurance, kind words, cards, flowers, the nurse, being indulged, opportunity to talk about how they feel, sentimental songs, family photos at the bedside, memories, feeling wanted, being needed, and warmth. Allow the family to visit (unless there is emotional stress). Natives of this auditorily sensitive Moon sign need calm and quiet! Soft music is healing and essential.

A happy stomach is the key to healing the Cancer Moon patient. "Comfort food," or Mom's fried chicken may not be best, but makes them happy. Dieting is difficult. Warm, nutritious home-made soups, made personally just for them, make miracles.

Although Cancer and Taurus Moon natives both love food, the approach varies. Cancer prefers what mother made, and is otherwise habitually selective; whereas Taurus Moon is our confirmed foodie of the zodiac, trying anything that smells good. Habitual eating can become a downfall for Cancer Moon folks, as they gradually lurch into a vitamin, protein or mineral deficiency, so typical of this sign. Do test any herbs or medicines first because this sign is famous for allergic reactions!

Never frighten the Cancer Moon patient. Use only positive suggestions, delivered in a cheerful, strong vocal tone. They will more readily accept the physician's authority than some other Moon signs. Therefore, never assent to negative questioning, i.e., "Doc, am I going to die?" Their subconscious will accept your verdict as reality, and obediently comply.

I remember with reverence old Doctor Shields in Portland who would place his hand on the shoulder of each patient as they exited his office, while stating in a firm, cheerful voice "You will get much better!" This is good practice for use with all patient types, although Cancer and Pisces are your most suggestive signs.

The sign Cancer is ruled by the Moon. It makes sense that those born with their Moon in this sign can experience extreme hormonal changes, fluidic fluxes and water retention during menses, with attendant changes of brain chemistry. The breasts are sensitive in this sign. Perhaps no Moon sign is as impacted by the Lunar phases as is Cancer. Be alert to "inexplicable" Moon-produced mood swings!

Remember, when it comes to Cancer Sun or Moon, a little kindness heals.

Leo Moon: Attention, Fun, Affection

The Leo Moon patient delights in pleasure, games, sunlight, watching favorite sports, the kids, hugs, lavish displays of affection, performing, drama, being the center of attention, receiving an excess of bright flowers and expensive gifts, their hamburger and beer, dancing (if possible), singing, visits from the gang, back rubs, laughter, being told they are the best (or the boss!), being needed, being alpha, being spoiled by the nurses, being made to feel powerful and in control (even while convalescing).

They readily enjoy the physician's visit, but may tell their doctor what to do! Few patients are more miserable when stuck in bed alone than are the Leo, or Leo Moon.

The emotions of love or anger strongly effect the physical heart for Leo Moon natives. Be alert for fluidic, or rhythmic heart changes and regard "broken heart" seriously. One often notes a pronounced weakness in the back muscles or spine.

Virgo Moon: Useful Work

Virgo Moon patients enjoy "programs," and will dutifully adhere to dietary and exercise regimes. They require, cleanliness, order, tidiness, quiet. They need to be useful and may refuse to quit work when they really should. The physician should be on the alert for orthorexia nervosa (self-starvation due to the pursuit of perfected food). Watch caloric intake for insufficiency. Anorexia nervosa is also common.

Assist these patients to relax, to let go (they often can't), to convalesce. It will be hard for them to accept help as they would rather serve others. They may need assistance with sleep.

Be astute with food and herb choices because this Moon sign gives sensitive intestinal organs and is prone to vomit up medicine (emesis). The upper digestive organs are "fussy," so start with low doses.

Nutritional remedies fascinate them, and typically their purse is a pharmacy. The physician needs to make sure they are not making themselves worse with an excess of supplements.

Libra Moon: Company, Balance, Beauty

The Libra Moon patient loves socially connecting with one person (at a time), flirting with the nurses, the spouse at the bedside, sweet treats, beauty, harmony, and a strong personal partner-like connection with their personal physician! Art (viewing) and beauty are as necessary to Libra as nutrients. Flowers are a must!

In long hospital stays, a dinner companion is essential. Natives of the Libra Moon may find solitude unbearable and need regular companionship to fully heal. Never allow them sit neglected in bed for protracted periods—they heal best when enjoying any activity that requires two (cards, chess, strolling, holding hands, etc.).

Negatively, this Moon sign is voyeuristic and addicted to movies, television, screens, etc. This can produce problems due to lack of exercise. The kidneys may be overactive, or sensitive. Consider strengthening the lumbar region, and tonifying the kidneys and ovaries.

Scorpio Moon: Involvement, Emotional Purging

These natives are entertained by medicine—so do tell them everything. They prefer flat out honesty, challenges, emotional intensity, herbal medicine, their favorite music or theater, intensely tasting or smelling herbal potions, emotional or physical releases and purging, intense therapies, and psychotherapy. Natural chemists, you might discover that they are self-prescribing herbs, or excessively dosing themselves.

Patients with this Moon sign incline to brew over the wrongs and betrayals they have experienced. Assisting with emotional clearance will greatly assist their recovery. Consider: Holly and Crab Apple Bach Flower Essences.

They crave purification. Be alert for excessive "cleansing" practices, laxatives, etc. Watch for excessive urination, nosebleed, uterine bleeding, endometriosis, candida. The uterus, genitals and bladder are sensitized.

Scorpio Moon patients are tough with themselves, are never sissies, and possess a strong will to regenerate themselves, but not yet equal to that of the Scorpio Sun! An active excretory system can assist, or impede health.

Sagittarius Moon:
Excitement, Stimulation, Knowledge, Adventure

Leg motion is a must; this sign finds it nearly impossible to "just rest." Natives of this Moon sign may require sleep aides! Staying prone is difficult, and in some cases, less necessary than for other signs.

If they cannot move, they become nervously agitated. Sagittarius Moon natives crave mental and physical excitement: study, learning, traveling (even a room change will help in the case of convalescence), and exercise. The convalescing Sagittarius Moon can be entertained for hours with webinars, documentaries, and a banjo.

Should claustrophobia, boredom or restlessness be displayed, allow them to convalesce outdoors in fresh air and sunlight. Panic attacks and hysteria are not uncommon maladies. Be on the alert for excessive caffeination, or conversely, alcoholism. Hot-dry-and-stimulated craves cold-wet-and-relaxing! Typically, they jack themselves up all day on caffeine, then attempt to relax with alcohol!

Often, they respond best to foreign therapies, exercise and diets. For instance, the Western Sagittarius Moon patient may be attracted most to Eastern health paradigms: yoga, t'ai chi, etc. Exercise and motion are essential. Be alert for later-life weakness in the hips or lower spinal nerves.

Capricorn Moon: Control, Order, Purpose

Natives of this Moon sign need discipline, regime, order. The environment must be neat (these patients are as tidy as those with Virgo Moon, if not more so). In fact, patients with this Moon sign can suffer from OCD.

Sudden intrusion is profoundly disturbing. Never surprise this patient with shots, probing or sudden hugs. Unexpected visitors may not be welcome (give them time to shape up). Describe all procedures in advance and during. Turn off the phones when they sleep. Allow them to remain in as much control over their bodies and space as is possible.

The physician should be on the alert for orthorexia nervosa (self-starvation due to the pursuit of perfected food.) Assist these patients to relax and let go. Relax the stomach and assist them to enjoy their food. Be astute with food, oil and herb choices because this Moon sign gives a dry mucus membrane and touchy gall bladder, and is quite prone to vomit up medicine (emesis).

Capricorn Moon natives have some tendency to fluid on the knee, weak knees, and light sensitive skin. Keep an eye on freckles, moles and sunburns. Capricorn Moon is common to females with some tendency to uterine fibroids or inadequate lymphatic action of the breast tissue; be vigilant. Typically, they make good patients, following their doctor's orders to the letter!

Aquarius Moon: Inspiration, Freedom

These patients require mental pleasure. They enjoy inspiring ideals, intellectual stimulus and deep studies. They have wide interests, and can entertain themselves for hours. However, they would rather die than suffer pain or nausea, and readily hurdle themselves into depressions. When in despair, the introduction of a great idea or philanthropic project will do wonders! If anything, they need to be part of a great work, something larger than themselves.

Patients of this Moon sign can sacrifice all personal joys if they feel they are serving a collective effort or higher cause (even if from bed). These people are wide-minded, enjoying great biographies, cartoons, astrology, anthropology, and all manner of odd topics. Humor and comedy can heal the Aquarian Moon patient, who often exhibits a highly developed sense of the absurd.

They are inventive! If convalescing, figure out what "great work" they can turn their hand or mind to.

To reiterate, Aquarius Moon natives are highly depression prone. They need light, movement, a higher purpose to live for, oxygen, minerals, vitamins, and above all, fresh air! Typically, they suffer a deficiency of one or more, and are prone to anemia. Often, they have lonely lives. It is good to inquire about their family or social life (if it exists).

This Moon sign native strongly tends to sub-oxygenation, low blood pressure and venous stagnation, especially at the ankles. This patient will probably demand to sleep with an open window, or will sneak out of bed to block off the room heater. Respect this preference or they will decline!

Provide warming stimulants, sunlight and circulatory support. They love salt, and need it. Vent heat can sicken them. Avoid carbonated beverages.

Judiciously used magnets, copper water or ionic therapies may work miracles. Think outside of the box and don't be afraid of following your healer's intuition!

Aquarius Moon patients enjoy friendly human contact—almost anyone will do! However, crowds, chaos and noise are draining to them. Few signs are more adversely effected by electromagnetic fields, so please protect them from EMFs and get them away from florescent lights! Traditionally, this Moon sign reacts strangely to chemical medicines and intravenous measures (as does Gemini Moon).

Natives of this Moon sign requires extra minerals, vitamins, oxygen and light. Mineral and magnetic therapies may resolve their tendency to massive and unexpected muscle spasm, anemia, blood insufficiencies, fatigue and depression. Do check for fluidic stagnation at the ankles, low blood pressure, foggy mind. Build the blood.

Pisces Moon: Faith, Peace, Tenderness, Love

These patients love sleeping, cuddling, and tenderness. Above all else, give quiet! It is torture for these natives to endure the constant bells, beeps and slamming doors of your average clinic. This sensitive and highly suggestible Moon sign responds best to kindness and reassuring words. However, they may require sequestering from close individuals who might be making them sick!

The psychic environment is more important for the Pisces Moon patient than almost anything else! The music, thoughts, television content should be monitored. Your Pisces Moon patient will scarce improve in a negative or scary psychic atmosphere! Conversely, vibrational remedies work more powerfully than for most other signs: homeopathy, flower essences, gem remedies, et cetera. Pisces works strongly through the unseen world!

Few signs respond as strongly to music. A diet of beautiful music is most helpful (ethereal, spiritual, sweet, romantic, harmonious genres). Patients with this Moon sign may require warming stimulants, enforced exercise and pep talks to keep going. Foot rubs are excellent! Watch for sloppy habits, lack of hygiene, carelessness with medicines, confusion, excess eating, and phlegmatic conditions.

Pisces Moon leans wet and atonic, requiring drying astringents, heart tonics and enforced exercise. There is some tendency to mineral and protein deficiency. The feet are extremely sensitive. Always work with, or through the feet with your Pisces Sun and Pisces Moon patients!

Natives of this Pisces Moon are acquiescing and patient when ill. They greatly enjoy being catered to, massaged, directed and dominated, and are pleased to leave the driving to you. Pisces Moon natives enjoy extreme closeness, and many thrive best with the affectionate help of a symbiotic lap dog. Pisces Sun and Moon live for love, and are notoriously oversexed.

In truth, the Pisces Moon patient requires more sleep than average, so allow it. Conversely, they escape through sleep. Today's "double Pisces" (Pisces Sun and Moon) client bore this rule out by conveying his roommate's complaints regarding his late sleeping hours, and long naps! The warming, drying stimulant herbs are a useful antipathetic treatment.

Never frighten the Pisces Moon patient. Use only positive suggestions, delivered in a cheerful, strong vocal tone. This is good advice for all patients types, but Pisces and Cancer are the most suggestible. And remember: happy feet make for a happy Pisces Moon native!

Chapter 12
PUBLIC HEALTH TRENDS

Have you ever wondered why your practice is suddenly deluged with knee cases? Or five patients on one day are desperate with migraines? Astrology is excellent at predicting daily, monthly and yearly public health trends!

Public Infection /Accident /Inflammation: Mars

The zodiac sign (Body Zone) that Mars currently transits through will correspond with a collective increase in accidents, inflammation, flus, muscle strains and infection within the body parts governed by that region! Although this varies considerably, Mars usually remains at least six weeks in any one sign.

Public Chronic Disease: Saturn

The zodiac sign (Body Zone) that Saturn currently passes through signals a collective increase in chronic problems, bone and structural issues associated with that bodily region. Saturn remains in any one sign approximately two and a half years.

Collective Fatigue: The South Lunar Node

The zodiac sign (Body Zone) of the current South Node will correspond with a collective increase in failure or fatigue within that bodily region, or mysterious viruses.

Mass Public Health Events: Eclipses

Eclipses strongly impact public health by indicating the bodily systems that are most collectively endangered. Eclipses will occur within one sign polarity for approximately one and one half years.

Think of these events as you would a long weather system! It behooves the wise physician to know if it is currently "the eclipse season of the heart," or "the eclipse season of the pancreas," et cetera.

The medical implications of eclipses through all twelve signs (Body Zones) with included calendar, can be accessed in my book *Eclipses and You.*

Chapter 13

TIMING FOR SURGERY AND TREATMENT

Do you want to reduce the potential for surgical and treatment error? Would you prefer to prevent medical suits? Although these useful rules don't cover all bases, they will assist you towards significantly reducing these potentials.

Note: Only the strongest rules, most easily grasped by beginners, are listed here. For an advanced, thorough discussion of surgical "dos" and and "don'ts," see *Medical Astrology: A Guide to Planetary Pathology, Chapters 22 and 23.*

When NOT to Perform Surgery or Commence Medication or Treatment.

This section is set in four subsections:

- Traditional Rules
- Patient Avoids (for surgery)
- Physician Avoids (reduce medical error!)
- Planetary Transit Influences in the Patient's Chart (more advanced)

TRADITIONAL RULES

1) Cut not with iron the body part governed by the sign (Body Zone) the Moon is currently passing through.

This is a very ancient rule, listed by Egyptian-born, Greek writer Ptolemy, in his seminal *Tetrabiblios*, published in 140 B.C.

The Moon pulls fluids to any bodily zone she passes through, heightening sensitivity in the region. Luna is also notably unstable and "moody" in influence. The chance of hemorrhage increases in the Body Zone cut when the Moon passes through its corresponding sign.

2) Surgery Type: Add to the body at the waxing Moon. Subtract from the body at the waning Moon.

For organ transplants, grafts, hip replacements, etc., it is best to use the waxing Moon. The period each month from new to full is "waxing."

For tumor, tissue, parasite, or pathogen removal, the waning Moon is vastly preferred. The period each month from full to new is "waning."

Most witches', new age, and farmer's almanacs show the dates of the new and full Moons each month. Jim Maynard's and Llewellyn's astrological calendars provide Moon phase, sign, and aspects (the relationships between the angle of the Moon and that of other planets).

3) Avoid full Moon and (maybe) new Moon.

Swelling of fluids and blood occurs, especially at full Moons, well known amongst nurses for their hemorrhagic effect. It is, therefore, unwise to have surgery at full Moons, too—within 24-48 hours!

New Moons are puzzling. Some writers feel the new Moon is somewhat strong for causing swelling and hemorrhage, whereas other writer's opine the reverse! The later note that the period approximately 45° (in time) prior to the new Moon (about three days time-wise), known as the Moon's early "balsamic" phase, is the best phase to use for avoiding hemorrhage!

This seems a good compromise for the avoidance of hemorrhage, but only in tissue removal procedures, most especially to limit the opportunity for regrowth of a removed tumor. The last quarter of the Moon would be best in these cases.

4) Avoid eclipses!

Unless unavoidable, perform no surgery, (or begin no onset of treatment) on eclipses (Solar or Lunar). This rule holds for more than just surgery. Eclipses act as triple-strength new or full Moons. In general, it is unwise to begin any course of chemical or homeopathic medicine during an eclipse or within 48 hours on either side of one. It is also a good idea to avoid the period between any two eclipses (one Solar and one Lunar), which are typically two weeks apart. I call this unpredictable period "between the waves."

Eclipses momentarily stop the flow of either Solar or Lunar light down their designated spinal channels, known in India as the Ida and the Pingala. The Ida, positioned at the left of the spine, channels Moonlight; and the Pingala, situated just at the right, channels sunlight.

At a Solar eclipse, the Sun's light is turned off then turned back on, creating an outage and then a surge of Solar force in the Pingala. A Lunar eclipse produces the same effect when Moonlight is turned off, then back on in the Ida. Polarity and sign is also involved, a subject dealt with at great length in *Eclipses and You.*

Eclipses appear to disturb electrical and magnetic energies of the body and the Earth in ways we scarcely understand.

Field Note: It is not wise to play Ben Franklin by taking a homeopathic medicine at the exact moment of eclipse totality.

One foolish friend decided to try a dose of homeopathic polio at eclipse totality, to see what might happen. He hardly lived to tell the tale, becoming instantly paralyzed and requiring a strong antidote.

Note: The more advanced rules below are for those with a little more astrological skill!

5) Avoid medical procedure when the Moon is passing over the patient's natal South Node or the current-time (transiting) Lunar South Node.

Once you know your symbols, you can find the sign position of your patient's South Node in his or her birth chart, or with the use of an ephemeris for his or her date and year of birth.

However, it requires greater skill to discern the half day or so when the transiting Moon is nearest to the current-time South Node (when little of productive worth occurs).

I'll reiterate the method for finding the South Node's sign from a previous chapter for those who just dropped in. First, find the position of the current North Node in your ephemeris. Yes, the North Node.

You will find that the current South Node is never listed. This is because you are "just supposed to know" that it will be exactly opposite in sign to the North Node. *(See "Opposite Signs/The Six Polarities" chart on page 36.)*

Once the Moon clears the sign of the current-time South Node by about 10°, you are now on safer ground to proceed, provided Luna is not now moving through the same sign as, and approaching the patient's natal South Node. A simultaneous good aspect from the Moon to current-time Jupiter or Venus can help allay this undesirable astrological condition.

Your handy pocket guide of daily planetary motion (Llewellyn's, Jim Maynard's, et cetera.) will inform you of the exact times of the Moon's "good aspects" to Venus and Jupiter with a small triangle symbol (for the trine) or asterix symbol (for the sextile). Perhaps this is the province of more advanced students.

PATIENT AVOIDS (FOR SURGERY)

1) Transit (current-time) Mars is conjunct your patient's natal South Node.

This means that transit (current-time) Mars is in the same sign as your patient's natal South Node, and very close by degree (orb). This is the worst time possible for surgery. Unless unavoidable, stay clear by several days.

2) Transit (current-time) Mercury is conjunct the patient's natal South Node.

This means that transit, or current-time, Mercury is in the same sign as your patient's natal South Node and very close by degree (orb). Expect mis-communications. This reliable aspect strongly warns of possible error in prescription, medical advice, or treatment. A diagnosis given at this time is so often wrong!

PHYSICIAN'S AVOIDS

(REDUCE MEDICAL ERROR!)

FOR PHYSICIAN'S PERSONAL BIRTH CHART

1) Avoid transit (current-time) Mars conjunct the physician's natal South Node.

This means to avoid transit, or current-time Mars in the same sign as the physician's natal South Node and therefore, very close. An astrologer may need to show you the date of exact "conjunction" or joining.

Physician should hang up an "on vacation" sign for about one week around this date. This conjunction comes around about once every two and a half years and lasts in great strength about a week, unless Mars decides to "station" here (slows down and stops before going retrograde). In that case, the aspect can last a month or more!

Years ago, an obstetrician hired me to find the dates in the calendar year when NOT to deliver or perform surgery. This period was always my suggested number one avoid! If you want to avoid surgical nightmares and consequential lawsuits, avoid this aspect! See the reverse aspect, below!

2) Avoid transit (current-time) South Node conjunct the physician's natal Mars.

This means that the transit, or current-time South Node is in the same sign as your natal Mars, and very close by degree (orb). Read the above section for the reverse aspect. If you are a surgeon, this period warns of a tendency for mistakes, reception of futile cases, or a decline in surgical acuity (usually temporary).

3) Avoid transit (current-time) Mercury conjunct the physician's natal South Node.

This means that transit, or current-time Mercury is in the same sign as the physician's natal South Node and therefore, very close. These are those few days where little things can go wrong with big consequences. Computers, phones, and all manner of communication devices may malfunction. Chances are high that you may give medical advice you will regret, or err in medical judgment or prescription.

If there was ever a time prone to faulty diagnosis, this is it! Keeping one's mouth shut is generally a wise. If possible, sign nothing. This is a great week to plan a little time off, as long as the office is in good hands. "When the cat is away, the mice will play."

This is a good time to check if the filing and accounting are in good shape, or conversely, a mess. You may have some surprises. Records get misplaced or lost. Patients cancel or forget their appointments, etc.

Hand acuity is off. See the reverse aspect, below.

4) Transit (current-time) Lunar South Node conjunct the physician's natal Mercury.

This means that transit, or current-time South Node is in the same sign as the physician's natal Mercury, and therefore very close to it.

Read all the above section for the reverse aspect. However, these effects last longer, and may have far reaching results. Fuzzy-mindedness or declining hand acuity are typical, (usually, but not always, temporary). Memory and general alertness slow down.

PLANETARY TRANSIT INFLUENCES
IN THE PATIENT'S CHART

This is a more advanced technique useful to skilled medical astrologers.

All planets, and most especially our "Big Four" cycle through our personal charts in various and complex cycles. Planets impart their influence by "planetary temperature" to any planet they conjoin or aspect. For a complete catalogue of transit effects, see *Medical Astrology in Action: The Transits of Health*.

Chapter 14
LUNAR TIMING TIPS FOR HERBAL MEDICINE

Here are "best in show" tips from a vast array of highly useful Moon lore for various and sundry medical purposes. These tips range in understanding level from layman to professional. (For more extensive material, see *Astrology & Your Vital Force, Chapters 6 and 7.*)

The Moon pulls magnetic energies and fluid to the Body Zone governed by the sign she passes through.

Luna spends approximately two and a half days in each sign, once each month. With few exceptions, no planet influences the current day as strongly as the Moon! To reiterate the header, Luna pulls magnetic energies and fluid to the bodily zone ruled by the sign through which she is currently passing. This ancient rule is so strong that you can actually observe this happening in many cases!

This astrological fact underlies the monthly and weekly cycles of many maladies. My friend, who was a little too fond of his wine, would invariably get "indigestion" each month as the Moon passed through Virgo, the sign of the liver (and also of his birth Saturn and South Node!). In astrological thinking, the Moon's transit through Virgo once per month hyper-sensitized his liver!

TRADITIONAL RULES

1) Do not give medicine when the Moon is passing through Earth signs (Taurus, Virgo, and Capricorn).

This is said to cause vomiting, especially if the Moon is also aspecting a "dignified" planet (a planet in signs it prefers) that is above the horizon line. Dr. Davidson adds that laxatives won't work at the Capricorn Moon!

2) Think twice before giving chemical medicine or intravenous procedures to persons who were born with their Moon in Gemini or Aquarius.

These folks are known to have extreme or inexplicable effects from chemical medicines because the nervous system is hyper-sensitive in these signs. Gemini governs the capillaries and Aquarius influences the veins.

3) Avoid the transit Moon in Aquarius for giving medicine, acupuncture, electrical treatment, etc.

This sign is famous for weird effects. If you don't believe me, have your hair cut when the Moon is transiting through this sign! Bizarre outcomes may occur because Aquarius appears to govern the little-known electrical system of the body. When the Moon moves through this sign, electrical activity picks up, creating blips, "surges" and "outages" of these little-known subtle currents.

4) **The Moon's transit of Water signs (Cancer, Scorpio, and Pisces) is the best time for the onset of herbal medicines or purgatives.**

Energy flows down and out. The excretory system is stimulated in Scorpio (bladder, nose, uterus, sweat glands, colon). Water signs are the most accepting, receptive, and diffusive... perfect for administering herbs. Laxatives, vermifuges, diuretics and diaphoretics taken on Scorpio Moons will act with doubled strength!

5) **For drying and warming: give medicine or treatment when the Moon is currently passing through Fire signs (Aries, Leo, and Sagittarius).**

The healer can use these Moon signs effectively to harvest, decoct or administer herbal medicines intended to heat and dry.

6) **For cooling and moistening: give medicine or treatment when the Moon is currently passing through Water signs (Cancer, Scorpio, and Pisces).**

Warning! Laxatives, diaphoretics and diuretics do double duty on the Scorpio Moon!

The healer can use these Moon signs effectively to harvest, decoct and administer herbal medicines intended to allay conditions of excessive heat or dryness. Cancer and Pisces are best for that purpose. Scorpio greatly relaxes the excretory system!

7) For casting, molding, setting, and astringing: use current-time Taurus or Capricorn Moon. Taurus is best for molding (dental molds, etc.). Capricorn is the most astringent of all signs.

However, we don't use Taurus Moon for dental surgery, or Capricorn for knee work. Virgo is the third Earth sign and useful for astringent needs, but too "mutable" (quick moving and fluctuating) for casting work. The transit Moon conjunct transit Saturn is potent for administering astringents and bone builders.

8) Fertility

Physicians, herbalists, and healers should all learn of the wondrous effectiveness of astrological fertility. There are ample books on this subject (google the "Jonas Method," or obtain the book about it entitled *Astrological Birth Control and How to Choose the Sex of Your Child*—a report on the work of Dr. Eugen Jonas by Sheila Ostrander and Lynn Schroeder.)

Dr. Eugen Jonas' fertility clinic operated for 11 years in what was then Czechoslovakia, with a proclaimed 80% success rate with both conception and gender preference, using astrological methods! My own experiences have corroborated his findings.

Health practitioners should know what all good farmers and breeders once knew, and many still do! Females of all species are more fertile when the Moon transits Cancer, Pisces, Taurus, and Scorpio (in this order of effectiveness). The following tips are for those with more advanced astrological skills.

There are manifold planetary conditions that lend themselves to increased fertility, or the reverse, infertility. I've written widely on this topic in other works, but will provide a few tips here for the more advanced reader.

The transit of Jupiter over a woman's natal North Node, or conversely, the transit North Node crossing over her natal Jupiter, heightens fertility. Transit of Mars in conjunction or good aspect with a lady's natal Venus, or transit of Venus conjunct her natal Moon, are also strong testimonies to assist successful conception.

Transits of Saturn or South Node reduce fertility when aspecting the natal Moon.

For male potency, we make the same observations when these planets aspect natal Mars. Transit of South Node conjunct natal Jupiter, or the reverse, (transit Jupiter over natal South Node) heighten the potential for miscarriage in pregnant women, if not remediated.

9) Nourishing the body—best timing

Identify the bodily zone you wish to strengthen or nourish. The twelve Body Zones ruled by each sign are provided for you in *Figures 1 and 2, Zodiacal Man, Chapter 4.*

When the transit Moon passes once monthly through the sign governing a specific Body Zone, or moves through one of its fellow signs of same element *(see next page)*, this causes slightly more blood, oxygen and thus, nutrients to flow to this region of interest. This effect is strongest for the sign that is actually governing the body zone concerned. Ignore this rule should the transit Moon be simultaneously passing over the patient's natal South Node or current-time South Node.

Sign Compatibility

Signs of the same element are
the most compatible with each other.

ELEMENT GROUPINGS

Fire: Aries, Leo, Sagittarius

Air: Gemini, Libra, Aquarius

Earth: Taurus, Virgo, Capricorn

Water: Cancer, Scorpio, Pisces

Chapter 15

DOCTOR-PATIENT COMPATIBILITY

For the more advanced student

This valuable section entails the comparison of specific planetary positions at birth, by sign, between the healer's chart and the patient's chart. This is not hard to do. All you need to discover is if the planet-pairs indicated in the following are in the same sign. If they are, then read the blurb!

For some, this technique may require a little help from some-one who knows how to compare two charts. This type of astrology is called "synastry." However, the rules here are simple. If you know your symbols, you should be able to follow along!

It is strange and marvelous to observe the powerfully uplifting effect of a physician whose birthday is exactly 'trine' his / her patient's! The trine angle (120° between any two planets on the seasonal wheel) is the most harmonious of all astrological aspects (angles).

All we are doing here is seeing if a select two planets are located in the same sign in the charts of both patient and physician. This is called a "conjunction."

The descriptions following are reliable in the great majority of cases, should the planets discussed be situated within 3° (numbers) of each other in the two compared birth charts. To discern if this is the case, just look at the signs, then the numbers listed beside the said planet in the birth chart. If you prefer, use the ephemeris and jot down the degree (number) of said planet given on the day and year of birth.

If the two planets mentioned in the blurb are in the same sign, and close by degrees, you have a match and can use the description. However, existing in a shared sign alone is good enough for the blurbs to hold. In working with patients, please also consider the physician's sections in the previous chapter on current-time conditions that are personally dangerous in a physician's or patient's birth chart for commencing medical procedure or surgery!

Example: Hypothetically, should the physician's natal Mars be at 2° Scorpio, and you have now found out that the patient's natal South Node is quite nearby at 3° Scorpio, take heed. The first point listed *(next page)* may be eerily relevant for this relationship. However, never ignore this ancient wisdom even if these planets are many degrees apart in the same sign. No doubt, there will still be some effect, though weaker.

I've selected the conjunctions (same sign pairings) that strongly work most of the time. However, no astrological rule exists without exception.

Have I left out important physician-patient aspects? Yes. There are, literally scores of them. I've selected the most reliable aspects occurring between two charts that are easiest for a novice to quickly see. The more advanced astrologer will be aware of many other combinations to avoid.

Harmonious signs, so essential to know, are listed, with illustration in the final section, entitled "Doctor-Patient Harmony."

PHYSICIAN-PATIENT DISHARMONY
(Avoids)
For the more advanced student

1) **The physician's natal Mars shares the same sign as the patient's natal Lunar South Node.**

This is one of the worst aspects a doctor or surgeon can have with his /her client. This warns of a grievous surgical error, with potentially severe ramifications. Strongest when the natal planets are within an orb (distance) of 0 to 5° of each other. Any healer seeing this should consider not taking the case, (especially if surgery is involved).

2) **The physician's natal Mercury is in the same sign as the patient's natal Lunar South Node.**

Another doozy. The doctor's advice will be probably be wrong for this person. Drug prescription may also be mis-applied. The patient may not hear correctly or understand important directions. Strongest at 0-5°.

3) **The healer's natal Saturn shares the same sign as the patient's natal Lunar South Node.**

The doctor's authority goes nowhere. This conjunction is particularly dangerous for surgeons implanting new bones, grafts, or replacement of joints. Long-term results are usually unfortunate.

However, in some cases, this aspect may indicate a karmic situation where the doctor or surgeon must correct a mistake from the past, or owes the patient a debt. Strongest at 0-10°.

4) Doctor's natal Sun is in the same sign as the patient's natal Saturn.

Not alway bad, but generally, the physician will become onerous to the patient, stultifying or scary. They will strongly feel his/her authority, but conversely, the healer may feel that the patient is bossing or controlling. The patient may associate the healer with either a dreaded or respected father figure in their life. They oppress the healer's vital force. Strongest effect at 0-10°. In most cases, avoid.

5) Physician's natal Saturn is in the same sign as the patient's Sun.

The physician is stultifying, authoritative or scary to the patient. The doctor is probably oppressive to their patient's vital force. The patient may become a chronic problem. If the aspect is close, avoid! In rare cases, this could turn into a suit.

6) Healer is born within 3 days of the patient's natal Lunar South Node.

Patient will tend to drain the doctor's energy, causing him/her to feel powerless, and lacking authority. Not always bad if well aspected by a mutual Sun-Sun harmony, or a happy Jupiter-Sun exchange (conjunction, sextile, trine). *(See next section on Physician-Patient Harmony.)*

7) Doctor's natal Mars shares the sign of the patient's natal Moon.

This is very strong within 0-5°. It warns of a patient's hyper-sensitive reaction to any penetrative medical procedure from the healer's hand; for example: shots, tubes, scopes, biopsies, or medicines. Healer must be very, very gentle with this person! In particular, the patient's stomach, breast, womb, brain, eye, and entire mucous membrane may hyper-react to any invasive procedure used by this healer.

This is also a very bad aspect between an obstetrician and a pregnant woman, producing a great chance of miscarriage, hemorrhage, and emergencies.

8) Sun sign disharmony *(disharmony of the vital force)*

For the more advanced student

Physicists observe that we are essentially made of sun-light, the photons streaming forth from the Sun. Astrologers observe that human beings are enlivened by 12 types of seasonal vital force, expressed as 12 Sun signs (the "zodiac signs"); 36 decans (ten-day divisions of these signs); four elements or densities of matter (Fire, Earth, Air, Water); and three modes, or rates of matter-in-motion (cardinal, fixed, and mutable).

In this paradigm, the physician's type and quality of vital force is as important to a patient's recovery as is any medication! I've written to great extent on this matter in my book

Astrology & Your Vital Force: Healing with Cosmic Rays and DNA Resonance. However, the simplest basics which most readers can readily learn are outlined here.

There exists an inherent energetic disharmony if the physician's natal Sun (the birth day degree) is closely square (90° angle on the season wheel) or quincunx (150° angle on the season wheel) to the patient's Sun (birthday degree). This means that the healer's specific type of vital force is disharmonious to the patient! This comes to bear when working with delicate persons, where every drop of vital force matters!

This does not necessarily mean that the two do / don't like each other, or even that they consciously feel this disharmony. The disharmony occurs on the deepest level and influences how the physician and patient exchange magnetism and prana (life force). Yes, it can be significantly reduced should positive inter-chart aspects intervene (see next section).

A more advanced ability to use an ephemeris is required to find the strongest incompatible dates by exact degree. For general purposes, you can use the sign lists given herein.

What about opposite Sun signs? This occurs when the healer is born opposite the patient on the seasonal wheel. These are generally not the best either, but in some cases provide a perfect needful magnetism to complement and balance the vital force of the patient.

What about same Sun signs? This is neutralizing and, while not bad, is not recommended.

"Squaring" Birthdays: Doctor and patient's Sun signs are 90° distant to one another *(see chart below)*. Generally, but not invariably disharmonious between healer and patient—friction, yet energy.

Exactly squared birthdays are the most abrasive, but not always. This is frequently seen in married couples! It could represent a needed fulfillment of a missing energy. A more advanced ability would be required to use an ephemeris to discover the dates positioned exactly 90° from any birthday). However, a general square by sign works, too, as shown below.

SQUARE BY SIGN

Aries / Cancer	Gemini / Virgo	Virgo / Sagittarius
Aries / Capricorn	Gemini / Pisces	Libra / Capricorn
Taurus / Leo	Cancer / Libra	Scorpio / Aquarius
Taurus / Aquarius	Leo / Scorpio	Sagittarius / Pisces

Quincunx: 150° distant (Use an orb of 3°.)

The vital force of the doctor cannot adequately fuel or influence the vital force of his/her patient.

This acts like a short circuit, potentially confusing or weakening to the patient. At the very least, it's like "dead air."

Should a patient whose birth day is at quincunx to the healer's own birth day fail to thrive under his/her care, it probably won't improve, and best to suggest another doctor.

A more advanced ability is required to use an ephemeris to discover the dates positioned exactly 150° and 210° from any birth date. However, the general signs work too, as given in the list that follows.

QUINCUNX BY SIGN

Aries / Virgo	Gemini / Scorpio	Leo / Capricorn
Aries / Scorpio	Gemini / Capricorn	Leo / Pisces
Taurus / Libra	Cancer / Sagittarius	Virgo / Aquarius
Taurus / Sagittarius	Cancer / Aquarius	Libra / Pisces

Opposite Birthdays: The "Polarities," 180° distant
(Use the "Opposite Signs" list below.)

This angle is either disharmonious, or, complementary and balancing! Each person's exact opposite birthday is their "half birthday." Many people marry their opposite sign. However, persons of opposite signs do not typically understand each other.

The dates in the year of exact opposition must be determined from an ephemeris (or from a comparison of actual birth charts). The opposite signs in general are listed below as the six traditional sign polarities.

OPPOSITE SIGNS / THE SIX POLARITIES

Aries – Libra	Cancer – Capricorn
Taurus – Scorpio	Leo – Aquarius
Gemini – Sagittarius	Virgo – Pisces

DOCTOR-PATIENT HARMONY
(See explanation and example page 119.)

1) The doctor's natal Mercury is in the same sign as the patient's natal Lunar North Node.

In general, the doctor's advice will benefit the patient and the doctor's medical judgment is correct. Selected medication is generally helpful. Effects are strongest at 0-5°.

2) Healer's birthday (natal Sun) is in the same sign as the patient's natal Jupiter.

This is singularly the best testimony of a fortunate connection. Provided no countering aspects intervene between the two charts, the physician is a blessing to this patient, protective to their health and life. Works well within an orb of 5°, though useful by sign alone.

3) Physician's natal Jupiter is in the same sign as the patient's natal Sun.

A positive testimony suggesting that this patient is good for the doctor! Effects are most reliable within an orb of 0-5°. Conversely, the physician is protective of the vital force of the patient.

4) The doctor's birth Sun is on the patient's natal Lunar North Node.

In a general way, the healer is a positive influence on this patient, provided there are no strong antipathetic inter-aspects between the two charts. *(See previous "Avoids.")* Works only in close orb of 0-3°.

5) Sun Sign Compatibility

It is essential for the healer's natural vital force to be fueling to that of the patient's vital force. This is best noted by comparing Sun sign elements in the manner presented below. This matter is so important that it comprises its own section.

Best Sun Sign Compatibility

Doctor and patient share the same Sun sign birth element (Fire, Earth, Air, Water), but not the same sign! *(See "Element Groupings," on page 118, and Figure 9, "Signs by Element Groups," on page 130.)*

A close "trine" occurs when two birth dates sharing an element are positioned approximately 120-125 days apart on the calendar. This is most fortunate. A more advanced ability to use the ephemeris is necessary to locate the exact dates that "trine" each other at precisely 120° apart. A few days on either side will provide a strong positive "complementary fuel" between the physician and patient! Complementary or "mating" fuel is a term coined the great healer William Gray.

If the doctor's birthday "trines" the patient's birthday in the manner above, then the healer's own innate type of vital force will be well harmonized to the patient's, creating the necessary "complementary fuel" (per healer William Gray). This works despite how well the healer likes / dislikes the patient! This fact is important to know when working with delicate persons, where every drop of vital force counts!

Harmony level of vital force, as shown astrologically, is one reason why one doctor futilely strives for months on a case that is instantly cured by another doctor who barely walks in the room! It is wise to consider doctor-patient astrological resonances. One doctor quickly cures a specific patient, while conversely, another doctor mysteriously produces a decline in this same person!

The healing effect a physician will have upon their "trine patient" works even if no particular affinity for the patient is felt! Also, the patient is far less likely to drain the healer!

Personally, I've corroborated William Gray's claim by witnessing three miraculous and instant healings occurring between healers and patients born on birthdays spaced exactly 120° away from each other. Students who study this phenomenon discover for themselves the great truth of Sun sign compatibility for all manner of human relationships. The ancients have bequeathed us a great key to healing!

I've written to great extent on this matter in my book *Astrology & Your Vital Force: Healing with Cosmic Rays and DNA Resonance*. The great healer, William Gray, also discusses this ancient knowledge and his own unique wisdom in his instructive book *Know Your Magnetic Field*. His biography is instructional reading: *Born to Heal*, by Ruth Montgomery.

Figure 9:

SIGNS BY ELEMENT GROUPS

(Master Key to Vital Force Harmony)

Signs of same element are compatible, providing healing "mating frequencies" to one another, (a descriptive term used by William Gray). The "masculine" Fire and Air signs are compatible, as are the "feminine" Earth and Water signs.

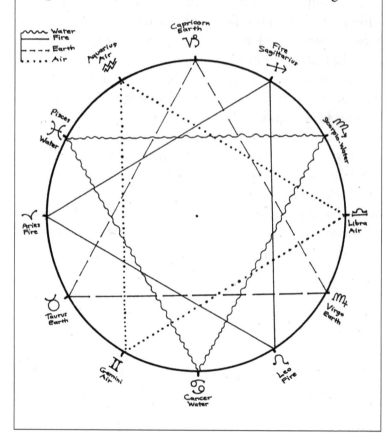

ADDENDUM

How to Read an Ephemeris

Much like anything else, in purchasing an ephemeris, you have choices. Ephemerides come by century! Current to this writing (2018) the most useful ephemeris spans 1950-2050. Most patients birth dates will happily fall within this period. Ephemerides are based on Greenwich Mean Time. This means that all planetary positions are calculated from London. You can choose between noon and midnight ephemerides.

The planetary symbols, provided for you in Chapter 3, and below, will be listed horizontally at the top of each month's page. The days of the month are listed vertically down the side of each months page.

Moving down each column, you will note little symbols for the astrological signs. You will find these same signs below.

Planetary and Sign Symbols

Planets	*Signs*
Sun ☉	Aries ♈
Moon ☽	Taurus ♉
Mercury ☿	Gemini ♊
Venus ♀	Cancer ♋
Mars ♂	Leo ♌
Jupiter ♃	Virgo ♍
Saturn ♄	Libra ♎
Uranus ♅	Scorpio ♏
Neptune ♆	Sagittarius ♐
Pluto ♇	Capricorn ♑
North Lunar Node ☊	Aquarius ♒
South Lunar Node ☋	Pisces ♓
Pars Fortuna ⊗	

When these "sign" symbols occur in the body of the vertical column, this alerts you that a planet has changed signs. As each sign contains 30°, planetary sign change ("ingress") always occurs when a forward moving planet has reached 29° 59'. A retrograde or backward moving planet (from Earth's viewpoint) changes signs at 0°.

In the vertical columns under each planet heading, at top you will sometimes see an "R" or "D." The "R" indicates a planet moving from forward to backward motion, or retrograde. The tiny "D" means the planet is turning back around and going direct. At these times the planetary energies are very focused indeed! In both cases, the planet appears from our standpoint on the Earth, to sit still, a condition that greatly strengthens said planet.

Malefic planets Mars or Saturn are most potent when moving backwards (i.e. "retrograde," symbolized in the column by "R") and just about to stop, standing still, as it were, from Earth's point of view (i.e. "station"). This is indicated with a "D" for "direct motion," appearing in the column, indicating that a planet is in fact, stationing, or "D," and now preparing to move forward again.

You will notice that for Saturn, there appears to be no motion at all for several days on either side of "D." At this time, he exerts a far more powerful influence than is normal, (as would any other planet). Noting "D" is especially helpful for charting the impact of the two "malefics," Mars and Saturn. Conversely, the two benefics, Venus and Jupiter are stronger too!

Conversely, when any planet is direct in motion, and slowing down to stop and reverse direction to now move backwards from the Earth's point of view, you will see an "R" in the column. Again, you will notice that the planet ceases all motion for some time on either side of the "R." In Saturn's case, this period will last for several days. As with "D", this period is far more potent for any planet.

Near "D" and "R," a planet's beams are focused on Earth in a very condensed manner. Think of holding your hand over a candle, and not moving!

EPILOGUE

In the face of enlightening facts and new discoveries, Western medicine chose to adopt an attitude of derision, disregard, and intolerance towards the whole of astrological knowledge. However, this was not always the case.

Throughout the European Renaissance, the newly emergent science existed in a brief, fruitful partnership with ancient planetary knowledge. Had this conflation continued, we would today enjoy Cosmobiological Departments in our hospitals, staffed with skilled professionals trained in the selection of safe surgery dates, the diagnosis of mysterious complaints, fertility, preemption of disease, doctor-patient compatibility, and the selection of medicines tailored to the individual's specific energetic portrait.

As the current Western medical model hungers for a more wholistic, and indeed, energetic approach, we now witness hundreds of young Western students applying each year to various accredited herbal and acupuncture schools. Many of these aspiring medical professionals are fascinated with the real science of medical astrology, and all it promises for suffering humanity. As this upcoming generation achieves maturity, so dawns a new medical era.

Perhaps we will finally achieve the lost promise of the Renaissance with the reinstatement of cooperation between ancient cosmobiological medicine, shorn of its less-desirable abuses, and modern, clinical medicine (equally shorn).

This author is not alone in her sentiment. The following quotes are extracted from the great French research scientist Michel Gauquelin, in his significant book, *Cosmic Clocks*, 1969.

"... The cosmos around us is neither changeless nor empty. The artificial satellites have shown clearly that space is filled with an infinity of corpuscles and waves buffeting our Earth, affecting everything that lives on its surface. In the thirty years or so that researchers have studied the matter scientifically, strange relationships between life and the universe have been discovered. Step by step, working its way in the shadow of established disciplines, a new science is emerging....

... The stage is now set for the last act of the cosmic drama, the most interesting and beautiful one. The rule of superstition ends here. A new science will replace the old cabala of cosmic dreams; it will help us assess man's true place in the riddle of the universe. We are indeed living through a turning point in human thought...."

Citation of Illustrations

Cover Illustration: "Sybil," from Johann Lichtenberger's Prognosticatio, printed in Venice by Nicolas and Dominico dal Jesus de Sandro, 1511.

Chapter 4: Zodiacal Man: Figures 1 and 2, Modern Zodiacal Man Charts anterior and lateral views, by Judith Hill.

Chapter 4: Figure 3: Homo Signorum- the man of signs, from Johann Regiomantus' Kalendarius Teutsch, printed by Johann Sittich, Augsburg, 1512.

Chapter 5: Figures 4: "Saturn in Gemini" by Judith Hill.

Figure 5: "Saturn in Leo" by Judith Hill.

Figure 6: "Mars in Gemini" by Judith Hill.

Chapters 6: Figures 7: "Mars in Leo" by Judith Hill.

Chapter 9: Allegorical drawing of the God Neptune, namesake of the planet, by Judith Hill.

Chapters 10: Small figure of man pointing to the Sun: unknown artist, Renaissance Europe.

Chapter 11: Small figure of man pointing to the Moon, unknown artist, Renaissance Europe.

Chapter 15: Figure 9: "Signs by Element Groups" (Master Key to Vital Force Harmony), by Judith Hill.

Facing "About the Author, page 146:" Depiction of the god Mercury with flute and caduceus by German engraver, Hans Burgkmair

WORKS BY THE AUTHOR

Books by Judith Hill

The Astrological Body Types, revised and expanded, Stellium Press, 1997.

An illustrated compendium of zodiac sign, planet, element and mode types, includes vast commentary and vocational attributions. Includes fascinating appendixes, including the research of Mars position in redheaded populations, medical nodes.

Medical Astrology: A Guide to Planetary Pathology, Stellium Press, 2005.

Complete A-Z guide. Medical information for Sun, Moon, planets and Lunar Nodes in all signs. Beginning to advanced material and rare topics (surgery, death, medical nodes). Includes one of the most thorough works on safe surgery timing. A "Dave's Top Ten" book by genre.

Astrology & Your Vital Force: Healing with Cosmic Rays and DNA Resonance, Stellium Press, Portland, OR, 2017.

The Sun's Master Cycle, William Gray's healing method, Sun Water for healing use, corroborative research of Buryl Payne, Ph. D, and others. Jyotish gem prescription methods and discussion of styles; zodiac-color theory and use; malefic houses and how to remediate; Moon-planet conjunctions for medicinal use; much more.

Medical Astrology in Action: The Transits of Health Stellium Press, Portland, OR, 2019.

For Natal and Transit Use. Forward by Matthew Wood. Mid-level to advanced material.

Includes descriptions of medical influence of transit Sun, Moon, planetary, and Lunar Nodes to the natal chart for all natal planets and both Lunar Nodes. Emphasis is on the conjunction and the quincunx.

Methods based on planetary energetics. Squares and oppositions discussed. Includes delectable Field Notes, Herbal Notes, Surgical Notes. Fabulously detailed.

The Lunar Nodes: Your Key To Excellent Chart Interpretation,
Stellium Press, 2010.
Includes "The Medical Nodes." Also: South and North Node in houses, signs; transit Nodes to natal planets; transit planets to natal nodes, thorough comparison of Eastern and Western traditions.
A "Dave's Top Ten" book by genre.

Eclipses and You: How to Align with Life's Hidden Tides,
Stellium Press, 2013.
Includes significant medical sections for eclipses in each sign.

Vocational Astrology: A Complete Handbook of Western Astrological Career Selection and Guidance Techniques,
A.F. A. Inc., 1999.
Winner of the Paul R. Grell "Best Book Award" for A.F.A., Inc. publications, 1999; A "Dave's Top Ten" book.

A Wonderbook of True Astrological Case Files,
(co-authored with A. Gehrz), Stellium Press, 2012.

The Part of Fortune in Astrology, Stellium Press, 1998.

Astroseismology: Earthquakes and Astrology, Stellium Press, 2000 (research compendium).

The Mars-Redhead Files, Stellium Press, 2000 (research compendium).

Mrs. Winkler's Cure, (by Judith Hill as Julia Holly), Stellium Press, Portland, Oregon, 2010.
Non violent fairy tales for the modern age. For ages 7-100.

Self-Study Courses for the Independent Student

MEDICAL ASTROLOGY 101
12 Module Course for the Independent Student
Available at: JudithHillAstrology.com
Optional: Final Exam and Certificate of Passage.
See: JudithHillAstrology.com

MEDICAL ASTROLOGY ADVANCED
Available Fall 2019

WEBINAR CLASS
"Astrological Medicine and Renaissance Herbalism"
with Matthew Wood and Judith Hill.
Available at:
The Matthew Wood Institute of Herbal Medicine.
See: JudithHillAstrology.com

Articles by Judith A. Hill

Judith Hill & Mark W. Polit, "Correlation of Earthquakes
with Planetary Placement: The Regional Factor,"
NCGR Journal, 5 (1), 1987.

Judith A. Hill & Jacalyn Thompson, "The Mars–Redhead
Link," NCGR Journal, Winter 88-89 (first published by:
Above & Below, Canada; Linguace Astrale (Italy); AA
Journal (Great Britain); FAA Journal (Australia).

"The Mars Redhead Link II: Mars Distribution Patterns in
Redhead Populations," Borderlands Research Sciences
Foundation Journal, Vol. L1, No. 1 (part one) and
Vol. L1, No 2 (part 2).

"Commentary on the John Addey Redhead Data," NCGR Journal, Winter 88-89 "Redheads and Mars," The Mountain Astrologer, May 1996

"The Regional Factor in Planetary-Seismic Correlation," Borderlands Research Sciences Foundation Journal, Vol. L1,Number 3, 1995 (reprint courtesy of American Astrology).

"American Redhead's Project Replication," *Correlation*, Volume 13, No 2, Winter 94-95.

"Octaves of Time," *Borderlands Research Journal*, Vol. L1, Number 4, Fourth Quarter, 1995.

"Gemstones, Antidotes for Planetary Weaknesses," *ISIS Journal*, 1994.

"Medical Astrology," *Borderlands Research Journal*, Vol. L11, Number 1, First Quarter, 1996.

"Astrological Heredity," *Borderlands Research Journal*, 1996.

"The Electional and Horary Branches," *Sufism, IAS*, Vol. 1, No 2.

"Astrology: A Philosophy of Time and Space," *Sufism, IAS*, Vol. 1, No 1.

"Natal Astrology," *Sufism, IAS*, Vol. 1, No 3.

"An Overview of Medical Astrology," *Sufism, IAS*, Vol. 1, No 4.

"Predictive Astrology in Theory and Practice," *Sufism, IAS*, Vol. 11, No 1.

"Esoteric Astrology," *Sufism, IAS*, Vol. 11, No 2, 3.

"Mundane Astrology," *Sufism, IAS*, Vol. 11, No 4.

"Vocational Astrology," *Sufism, IAS*, part 1 and 2, Vol. 111, No 1, 2.

Articles by Judith Hill (continued)

"Astro-Psychology," *Sufism, IAS*, Vol. 111, No 3, 4.

"The Planetary Time Clocks," *Sufism, IAS*,
Vol. 4, No 1, 2, 3, 4.

"Astrophysiognomy," *Sufism, IAS*, Vol. 4, No 1, 2.

"Spiritual Signposts in the Birth Map," *Sufism, IAS*,
Vol. V, No 2, 3.

"The Philosophical Questions Most Frequently Asked of the
Astrologer," *Sufism, IAS*, Vol. 5, No 4, Vol. 6, No 1, 2.

"Music and the Ear of the Beholder,"*Sufism, IAS*, 1999.

"The Astrology of Diabetes," *Dell Horoscope*, October 2003.

"A Life Time of Astrology," published interview with Judith
Hill, by Tony Howard, *The Mountain Astrologer*, Nov-Dec,
2010.

"Great Earthquakes of Northeastern Honshu (1900-2011):
A Planetary Portrait," *The Mountain Astrologer*, 2011.

"The Astrology of Depression," *Skyscript*, 2017.

"The Lost Secrets of Renaissance Medicine," *ANS,
(Astrological News Service)* 2017.

BIBLIOGRAPHY AND SUGGESTED READING

Bhattacharjee, Shivaji, *Astrological Healing Gems*, Passage Press, Salt Lake City, UT, 1990.

Beckman, Howard, *Vibrational Healing with Gems*, Balaji Publishing House, Pecor, NM; Gyan Publishing House, New Delhi, 2000.

Bhattacharya, A. K. and Ramchandra, D. N. *The Science of Cosmic Ray Therapy or Teletherapy*, Firma KLM Private LTD, Calcutta, 1976.

Bhattacharyya Benoytosh, M.A., Ph.D., revised and enlarged by A. K. Bhattacharya, *Gem Therapy*, Firma KLM Private LTD., Calcutta, India 1992.

Brown, Richard, S. G.I.A., *Ancient Astrological Gemstones & Talismans*, A.G.T. Co. Ltd., Publishers, Bangkok, Thailand, 1995.

Blagrave, Joseph, *Blagrave's Astrological Practice of Physick*, London, 1671, edited by David R. Roell, Astrological Classics, 2010.

Cayce, Edgar: *See "Winston"*

Cornell, H.L. M.D., L.L.D., *The Encyclopaedia of Medical Astrology*, Llewellyn Publications and Samuel Weiser, Woodbury, MN, 1972.

Cramer, M.s., Diane, *How to Give an Astrological Health Reading,* The American Federation of Astrologers, Inc., 2005.

Davidson, William, *Davidson's Medical Lectures,* edited by Vivia Jayne, The Astrological Bureau, Monroe, NY, 1979.

Davison, Alison, Metal Power, *The Soul Life of the Planets*, Borderland Sciences Research Foundation, Garberville, CA,1991.

Grey, W. E., *Know Your Magnetic Field*, Christopher Publishing House, Boston, MA, 1947.

Heindel, Max, *Astro-Diagnosis, A Guide to Healing*, 11th edition The Rosicrucian Fellowship, Oceanside, CA, 1928.

Jain, Manik Chand, *The Occult Power of Gems*, Ranjan Publications, New Delhi, India, 1988.

Jansky, Robert Carl, *Modern Medical Astrology*, AstroAnalytics Publications, Van Nuys, CA, 1978.

Johari, Harish, *The Healing Power of Gemstones in Tantra*, Ayurveda, Astrology Destiny Books, Rochester, VT, 1988.

Kapoor, Dr. Gouri Shanker, *Gems & Astrology*, Ranjan Publications, New Delhi, India, 1985.

Kollerstrom, Nick, *The Metal Planet Relationship*, Borderland Sciences Research Foundation, Garberville, CA, 1993.

Light, Phyllis, *Southern Folk Medicine*, North Atlantic Books, 2018.

Millard, Margaret, *Case Notes of a Medical Astrologer*, Red Wheel, Weiser, Boston, MA, 1980.

Montgomery, Ruth, *Born to Heal: The Amazing True Story of Mr. A. and the Astonishing Art of Healing with Life Energies*, Montgomery, AL, 1973.

Nauman, Eileen, *Medical Astrology*, DHM, Blue Turtle Publishing, Cottonwood, AZ, 1982.

Payne, Buryl, Ph.D., "Apparatus For Detecting Emanations From The Planets," The Journal of Borderlands Research Sciences, Vol. XLVI, No. 6, Nov-Dec 1990, pp 7-11.

Popham, Sajah, *Evolutionary Herbalism*, North Atlantic Books, California, 2019.

Ridder-Patrick, Jane, *A Handbook of Medical Astrology*, Penguin Books, London, NY, 1990.

Saha, N. N. Stellar, *Healing: Cure and Control of Diseases Through Gems*, Sagar Publications, New Delhi, 1976.

Simmonite, W. J., *The Arcana of Astrology*, North Hollywood: Symbols & Signs, 1977.

Tansley, David V., D.C., *Radionics & the Subtle Anatomy of Man*, Health Sciences Press, Bradford, Devon, Holsworthy, England, 1972.

Starck, Marcia, *Healing with Astrology*, Crossing Press,1997.

Tarnas, Richard, *The Passion of the Western Mind*, Ballantine Books Edition, 1993, by arrangement with Harmony Books, a division of Crown Publishers, Inc, NY.

Uyldert, M., *Metal Magic: The Esoteric Properties and Uses of Metals*, Turnstone Press Limited, UK, 1980.

Westlake, Aubrey T., *The Pattern of Health*, M.D., Shambhalla, Berkeley and London, 1973.

Winston, Shirley Rabb, *Music as the Bridge*, based on the Edgar Cayce Readings, A.R.E. Press, Virginia Beach, VA, 1972.

Wood, Matthew, *The Practice of Traditional Herbalism*, North Atlantic Books, Berkeley, CA, 2004.

Wood, Matthew, Francis Bonaldo, and Phyllis Light, *Traditional Western Herbalism and Pulse Evaluation*, Lulu Publishing, 2004.

Wood, Matthew, with David Ryan, *The Earthwise Herbal Repertory*, North Atlantic Books, Berkeley, CA, 2017.

Yogananda, Paramahansa,*The Bhagavad Gita, Royal Science of God-Realization*, verse 29 p. 634, Self-Realization Fellowship, Los Angeles, CA, 1996.

Young, Arthur M., *The Geometry of Meaning*, A Merloyd Lawrence Book, Delacorte Press, 1976, and *The Reflexive Universe*, Robert Briggs Associates, Mill Valley, CA, 1976.

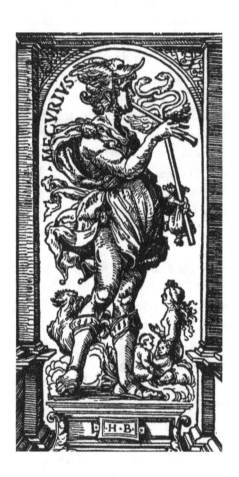

ABOUT THE AUTHOR

Judith Hill is a second-generation, and lifetime consulting astrologer, having performed over 9,000 readings to date. She is also an astrological researcher, teacher, publisher and award-winning author of thirteen books. These include her medically relevant titles:

Medical Astrology: Your Guide to Planetary Pathology;
Astrology & Your Vital Force: Healing with Cosmic Rays and DNA Resonance;
Medical Astrology for Health Professionals
and the classic *The Astrological Body Types.*

Some of her writings have been translated into Russian, Vietnamese, Italian, Lettish and Arabic.

Hill is a Chartered Herbalist with *The Dominion Herbal College.* Judith Hill and Matthew Wood created the Webinar course "Astrological Medicine and Renaissance Herbalism" through *The Matthew Wood Institute of Herbalism,* produced by Tara Baklund.

Judith created the course "Medical Astrology 101" for the independent student and later introduced traditional Western medical astrology to students in Szechuan, China (2017-18).

Hill conceived and co-produced the first exclusively medically oriented astrology conferences in Portland, Oregon:

"Medical Astrology Day," (with OAA board members, M. Neuner and S. Scott) and obtained sponsorship from AFAN (1992); and "Medical Astrology Day," with the assistance of D. Tramposh (2008).

She later created and produced the annual "Renaissance Medicine Conference"© in Portland, Oregon, pioneering the conflation of medical astrology and herbal-alchemical conferences in the USA.

One of Judith's contributions to medical astrology is her original documentation of the comprehensive medical and physical implications of the Lunar Nodes through both their natal and transit conjunctions to each planet and sign; and also by detailing the medical impact of eclipses through each zodiac sign and in aspect to planets.

Judith served as the Educational Director for the San Francisco Chapter of *The National Council of Geocosmic Research*. She worked for ten years in the statistical study of astrology, receiving an unsolicited research grant from *The Institute for the Study of Consciousness*; and produced two widely acclaimed research compendiums: "The Mars-Redhead Files" with Jacalyn Thompson, and "Astro-Seismology" with Mark Polit.

As a pioneer in astro-seismology and astro-genetics, she founded *The Redhead Research Project*; Stellium Press ("for stellar minds"), and San Francisco's first "NCGR Research Day" in the late 1980s. Near this time she briefly worked as an astrological research project assistant for the renowned physicist Arthur Young in Berkeley, California, and assisted KCBS radio's Editorial Director Joan Margalith with her pioneering *Infinity* radio show.

As a "road tested" astrologer, Hill successfully matched five charts to five biographies in a 1989 NCGR-sponsored skeptic's challenge, and successfully predicted (and pre-published) the magnitude, general time and location of California's famous "Loma Prieta" Earthquake.

Her breakthrough astrogenetic research was featured on Television's syndicated program *Strange Universe*.

Additionally, she segregated and documented the impact of eclipses according to their nodal polarity (North vs. South Node eclipses, for both Solar and Lunar eclipses); and published possibly the first eclipse calendar for astrological use, inclusive of stated nodal polarity. Hill also documented the potential physical and health effects of most transits in her pioneering work *Medical Astrology in Action: the Transits of Health* (2019).

In the 1980's, Hill authored what may be the first serious column on real astrology outside of the popular press, entitled "Astrology, a Philosophy of "Time and Space" for *Sufism Magazine*.

Judith has lectured widely for multiple conferences, groups, podcasts, radio and television shows both inside, and outside of the astrological world. A biographical interview with Judith by noted producer and astrologer Tony Howard was featured in the December, 2010 issue of *The Mountain Astrologer Magazine*.

In her spare time, she is a professional musician and vocalist in multiple genres, producer, sculptor, teacher, tree advocate, illustrator, "roadside anthropologist," and Jewish heritage historian.

JudithHillAstrology.com

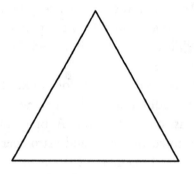